WHO LIVES, WHO DIES
WITH KIDNEY DISEASE

WHO LIVES, WHO DIES
WITH KIDNEY DISEASE

MOHAMMAD AKMAL/
VASUNDHARA RAGHAVAN

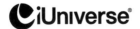

WHO LIVES, WHO DIES WITH KIDNEY DISEASE

iUniverse books may be ordered through booksellers or by contacting:

iUniverse
1663 Liberty Drive
Bloomington, IN 47403
www.iuniverse.com
1-800-Authors (1-800-288-4677)

ISBN: 978-1-5320-5297-2 (sc)
ISBN: 978-1-5320-5298-9 (e)

Print information available on the last page.

iUniverse rev. date: 07/06/2018

Contents

The most important thing in illness is never to lose heart.

— Nikolai Lenin

Introduction

Dealing with illness, particularly major diseases, has always been a challenge. How it affects a person is defined by factors such as physical condition, family circumstance, economic background and personal attitudes. Patients relying heavily on medical experts' advice, find it easier to manage the disease while others who are experimental cause medical professionals' great concern as they increase their exposure to unwanted diseases and face needless complications. Evaluating patients based on observing their psychological behavior measures well, as it brings humanness to the forefront as against using predetermined benchmarks that makes no differentiation based on patient's individual needs.

With chronic kidney disease growing in numbers and existing skew in ratio of physicians to patients, there is growing concern for physicians as well as the community that every patient is not getting enough attention. Physicians in Nephrology are looking at ways to address this limitation by developing new sustainable models of health care, conducting training programs for graduates increasing awareness of the disease amongst public and programs like early detection to reduce burden of the disease.

Reviewing patients and their disease management has shown many people have been successful in managing to survive the disease against all odds, and rightly they may be considered fortunate. Unaware of consequences of being negligent, many people make huge mistakes and land in situations that reduces chances of recovery making them unfortunate. At a time when understanding and sympathy would help in healing, sometimes family and friends get critical making the person feel guilty and slowly the patient withdraws from social life. Over time patients choosing to remain isolated has only developed fear in public mind of the disease and truth has remained shrouded. Physicians are continuously reviewing and formulating changes in their approach to patient care so alarming levels of critical conditions are minimized.

Complexity of chronic kidney disease is vastly undermined in all parts of the world. Our attempt through this book is to share stories of people who experienced the disease, challenged it; some of them lost the battle while some others created history. Through narrative of individual stories readers will realize the deeper issues that place patients on tenterhooks. For families of patients there will be an opportunity to find new areas they need to understand about psychological issues faced by their kith and kin. For the very first time, readers will walk through those dark roads that health could take, placing huge challenges that could even be at their door, if early signs are ignored. As for the medical fraternity there's another reminder to appropriately raise alarms for benefit of communities.

The book will engage a reader with heart-warming stories and gradually move in subsequent chapters to some critical information so it becomes a good learning experience. For some it could be first time information on basic knowledge about the organ and it's functioning. Some stories puts speculation at rest by focusing on lifestyle changes that helps in better health management. Some interesting guidance from patients comes through story's narrative and we have given some first level tips that could change mind-set of patients and families.

In 2006, I met Vasundhara Raghavan, when her son Aditya Raghavan was under my care. After a kidney donation in 1999 she developed a deep understanding of the disease and showed considerable interest in kidney related research studies. This led to our conversations around raising awareness on chronic kidney disease. Interesting developments led to two books being released, with our belief and conviction that the disease needs to seen from the patient's perspective. Vasundhara is actively advocating for awareness of chronic kidney disease management including dietary issues on Facebook support groups and doing considerable work in India.

This book and our earlier publication, *Shades of Life, Sublime Joy is in Living* attempts to show that a patient's life is beyond dialysis and transplant. Reality is that diet, exercise and medications play a huge role in disease management. Life is filled with anguish, uncertainty and intense suffering for patients and their families. Living and existence may have different connotations but for people dealing with kidney disease, the stark difference is so huge that it becomes difficult to demarcate the two. Comfort comes through community's appreciation of the disease, understanding of patient's pain and supporting them to face chronic kidney failure with courage.

Honoring patient confidentiality, respecting sensitivities of a few, readers will notice individual identities are safeguarded. With consent of those specially interviewed for this book, their names and photographs are published. All the stories will resonate with trials and tribulations of people from different walks of life. But cost implications of treatments for chronic kidney disease will stand as a single significant differentiator. I am sure in future meeting a person with chronic kidney conditions will touch an emotional chord.

Mohammad Akmal, MD
Professor of Medicine, Keck School of Medicine,
University of Southern California

Kidney Lives

Today over 7 billion human beings occupy planet earth and the figure grows each minute. Human lives have a definitive purpose to live as characters molded by environmental influences powered by an intuitive mind. Each soul is captive to an exclusively charted path that could cross paths with others in their journey.

Was a pure and perfect life just a creation of an imaginative mind? Or was such a mystical existence witnessed before and undergone sea change?

Legend goes that the first human existed several hundreds of thousands centuries ago. They walked through green lands, enjoyed the clear blue sky above, tasted nectar in the sparkling water that gurgled down as a bountiful cascade, meandering over stretches of plains, while solid rock structures symbolized impregnable toughness.

Caught by fantasy of such magical past one wonders when and how imperfection entered the planet's orbit. Gradual conquests by an unworthy character possessing extraordinary manipulative skills, driven by personal ambitions could have spurred creation of a new domain where greed of a silent, purposive intruder systematically planted thoughts then actions, to endanger existence of the innocent breed.

But the air, wind, sun, water also worked as an undercurrent to stretch things further, adding many compulsive distractions mesmerizing mankind. World was no longer fantastical beauty, but it became real where mankind exercised his heart and brain to fathom the turbulence ahead. At each bend human beings used superior intellect to overcome and squash it. But there was much more that awaited them.

Through the pages of this book we will look at a particular hurdle faced by human race. Kidney disease got recognized as an ailment that affected people in different ways. How, how much, how well it was managed will be seen over time. People who became instrument to overcome the hurdle lived in this universe at some point of time. They gave us something surreal, something that their passionate ways brought about changes in life and living.

Early days

Tide was forever rising and waning. With that people's lives saw dramatic swings of happiness and despair. For the ones with ability to smile and take life in their stride life was enjoyable. They fought challenges; achieved goals by raveling difficult situations through experimentation, speculating cause for success and failure with equal interest. But some of them belonged to a community who experienced fear, saw adversity and were confounded by an impenetrable wall that many others managed to conquer with persistence.

What was this invincible power that drove people to a madness, one wondered? Nothing was as clear as crystal. Nothing was heard, not even a whimper. Nothing could be understood. All in all it was mysterious. It had pain and uncertainty crouching in the shadow waiting to pounce unwarranted.

The first time when a person confronted it, was he vowed into silence? Why is it under a thick shroud of darkness? Was there anything that was paranormal? Did the earliest incident leave the person mesmerized? Was it considered as the devil himself, large and daring?

It is said that as early as 100 AD it was first seen, noticed and recognized. Stories of events at Roman baths made rounds. Some people soaked long hours and enjoyed a bath immersed in a great body of water. It was discovered that it was a build-up of urea. If one soaked in baths the toxicity was removed. It was believed to be as effective as today's dialysis.

Then in 1500 AD a fully recorded case of Stefan Bathory, King of Portland was later matched with symptoms of Polycystic Kidney Disease. One can safely say that such evidence got recorded since a State Head of a Kingdom showed some weird health conditions. Apart from attracting curiosity, some questioning minds possibly wondered on what caused the disease.

The history of urinary tract stones began with history of civilization. In 1901, an English archaeologist E. Smith detected a bladder stone from a 4500-5000 year old mummy in El Aimash, Egypt. Furthermore, treatment for stones had been described in ancient Egyptian medical writings from 1500 BC. In 1807, an English physician Richard Bright described a disease characterized by edema (swelling of body); presence of albumin (protein) in the urine and high blood pressure and this disease was name after him as "Bright's disease".

It isn't an overstatement if one is said to feel marooned, when unceremoniously a urine-producing organ decides to shut down, either completely stopping urine production or began leaking protein in urine. The body enters a totally uncomfortable state of being. Breathlessness, headache, nausea, loss of appetite for food or water, body swelling and back pain are some promptings bringing to the forefront uncertainty of life.

The kidneys rank as one the most important organs; they produce urine, eliminate waste products, and synthesize important hormones. Surprisingly, people generally refer to the fullness of the bladder when they have to go to the bathroom and remember the kidney only when they cannot urinate. The Latin term *renes* is related to the English word reins, a synonym for the kidneys in Shakespearean English. The kidneys, always used in the plural (*kelayot*), are mentioned over 30 times in the Bible. In the

Pentateuch (the first Jewish and Christian scriptures), the kidneys are cited 11 times in the detailed instructions given for the sacrificial offering of animals at the altar.

Kidney is an organ present in many animals, and in humans they are located behind the abdominal cavity near the middle of the back below the rib cage. Majority of the people possess two kidneys, one on each side, while in rare cases some have to live with one kidney (being born with one or losing one of them either surgically or in an accident). Occasionally, people are born with one or both small and poorly functioning kidney/s.

This bean shaped organ may each be as small as a fist and is blessed with a million functioning units called nephrons, which are the key performers in the kidney's function.

In humans the kidneys perform very important function but are sometimes victimized by diverse conditions and disorders. These medical conditions may be congenital or acquired. Some disorders that could cause chronic damage to this organ are the diabetes, hypertension, chronic glomerulonephritis (inflammation of small blood vessels in the kidney), chronic tubule-interstitial nephritis (damage to the tubules and tissues that surround them called interstitial tissue), polycystic kidney disease, and systemic lupus erythematosis, among many others.

For people affected by the disease, annual treatment of CKD runs into billions. In some economically advanced countries, patients have the opportunity to decide between hemodialysis and peritoneal dialysis. Furthermore, some eligible patients receive kidney transplantation. In US most kidney transplantations are cadaveric, needing a few years of wait time. Less frequently, some lucky individuals receive a kidney from a relative, and others occasionally get it from an unrelated donor. All these treatment modalities are expensive and are not readily available in most developing countries and rationed in the countries with emerging economies.

How likely will it be that one will recognize the onset of the disease and act quickly! It is widely known that reaction to the disease is generally slow and body's slowing down comes many a time with an element of surprise, bordering on a state of shock.

How much of this has it changed in the second decade of the 21st century?

Kidney failure is widely acknowledged as serious, but today it becomes the 9th disease causing more deaths. Though the course of the disease has travelled quickly, breaking many barriers, conquering many turbulent waters, but there is a growing quest for squashing the finer, microscopic elements that keeps it in the realm of "life-threatening disease". The balance can tip between life and death with even a miniscule dietary change.

We have come a long way since early reporting. Transplants have improved; Dialysis treatments are customized meeting levels of comfort and convenience, providing a good lifestyle. Developmental work improved dialysis machines to bring greater efficiency in dealing with toxicity and constantly medications are improved to minimalize side effects. However, treatments continue to be cumbersome and expensive. Care providers have found new ways to spread information so early detection is possible. Many organizations are focused on conducting preventive camps.

The patient however, continues to remain deeply involved in finding ways to survive. None of the work done by medical fraternity has much significance. Chronic kidney disease has treatments, but there's no cure.

Mohammad Akmal, MD
Professor Emeritus
Keck School of Medicine
University of Southern California
Los Angeles, CA

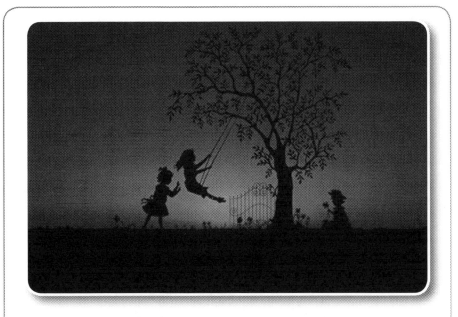

RACING TO WIN- MALU NARA INDIA

"Malu...I am sure to win. Watch me...just how every minute I am reaching closer to the sky... Here I go!"

With every ounce of energy, I pushed hard on the gravel. My legs were longer than hers; I was plump, more energetic, and more confident. She was my age, smaller and fragile. At that point it didn't bother me that I was flaunting my superior physique and taking full advantage of it.

It was a warm, summer mid-day, the air hung with happiness as school was closed and vacations had just begun. To set the mood and the whole picture perfect, the birds chirped endlessly as if a huge forum of speakers were involved in a cheerful debate. I simply loved the garden and the green trees hanging low, swaying with the breeze, in the process losing some precious flaming red Gul Mohair flowers.

In my heart, that for some mysterious reason Malu was in awe of me. Her non-communicative ways and soft manner clashed with my overpowering manners, but her docile ways somehow suited me. Who likes to handle a tyrant!

Now as I had made my mind to win, I busied myself, focusing on pumping my energy to reach my target.

Every time I kicked the mud and moved up I could see the blue skies and a bird flying by. It was a happy thought sitting on the rough, hard wood dreaming of winning while Malu sat tight on her swing in a red and white polka dress, making little effort to ride high. I could feel my knee-length pink and blue summery, floral dress floating merrily as if in celebration.

While I enjoyed myself, laughing mirthfully from her side, there was no sound except the creaky noise of the swing, pleading to get some lubrication.

Even as I was busy and fully engrossed in play I saw a manservant, rushing towards us with beads of sweat on his forehead...

"Come...come...Master is calling you. Some bad news..."

He was breathless and with some agitation he pulled the swings clumsily using full force to bring them to a rude halt. Malu seemed very eager to leave her perch though she walked at a slow pace, without even bothering to look back at me.

I was unsympathetic and thought, "What an end to this game! I was surely the winner!" But, surprisingly I never drew courage to pass rude comments to her.

Boredom set in as I strolled back to the house, kicking mud as if still in play and angry to be forced to head back to the house.

Malu's house was a huge mansion standing proud and majestic occupying a very large green, wooded area. Red roofed, with two robust chimneys emitting smoke when the house was filled with guests. Today there was a thin line of smoke making way to the sky. As it was nearly lunchtime I wondered if anything exciting would be served for lunch.

Looking up again I inspected the house closely, with admiration and hoped that my Dad would buy one such home with a sprawling garden. I would ask Dad to make a small playhouse on the edge where I could sit for hours, painting or playing monopoly with my friends. I could even read a book with a cushion tucked under my arm. A mini ladder stacked with some snacks and drinks would make it complete summer retreat.

Taking a deep breath I realized this would remain a pipe dream! No chance of ever becoming real!

As I drew closer, as if the winds had swept it clean the verandah looked empty and forlorn. Entering the patio I had the chilling feeling of being left alone. A huge silence shrouded the house. My palms closed in a clasp, wet and sticky as I stood there for a moment feeling the lonely sound of silence.

I entered and saw the front drawing room had a fan furiously swirling away. I saw the women were quiet; faces looked lost and indifferent, as if stranded on an empty road that led nowhere. Suddenly they busied doing trivial things. The stillness was scary, as if time was held back, even though the huge grandfather's clock clicked away loudly.

In normal times this room was the busy coffee room. One associated it with strong aromas of freshly brewed coffee and an array of freshly prepared snacks. Some days, the garden tables were laid with picnic basket, from where Aunt Laxmi and Mom, would dig up boxes with exciting food. Oh, what fun those times were!

But now I noticed everything was starkly different. I saw the room ripped of all happiness, paled down to look drab and insignificant.

Mom pulled me roughly by my forearm and whispered between tight lips, "There's some bad news. Sunder died in the cinema house a few minutes back."

Then looking straight into my eyes, with her pointer finger held tight on her lips she said, "Hush...."

I looked into hers, suddenly large with fear and anguish. I was quiet. Not daring to do or say anything!

Magically the sun took shelter behind thick clouds. Darkness cast over the summery house with teak doors thrown open, ventilated high ceilings that under normal circumstances made the rooms airy and comfortable, but now even the air was heavily doused into silence.

Everyone looked sullen with no trace of warmth.

This tense atmosphere drew the worst in me. I felt claustrophobic. On tiptoes I walked to the window to take refuge behind the heavy curtains. At least the happiness of the world outside could cheer me.

In the garden the swing was slowing down and I knew in sometime it would come to a complete halt. Suddenly a car lunged forward out of the porch and caught up speed. Dad and Malu's father were seated in the rear seat, while the seat beside the driver, was occupied by an unfamiliar person.

Their faces wore a mask of solemnity.

As if perfectly timed, as soon as the car zoomed out of sight, Aunt Laxmi burst out aloud, tears streaming down her cheeks and Mom did all she within her means to pacify her. Aunt ranted, "My poor child...he was just eighteen years old..."

Mom agreed with her and added words to similar effect.

"What harm did he bring about? Why is he punished?"

Everyone tried hard to console and soothe Aunt Laxmi. But she was inconsolable. My sisters were swarming around Aunt Laxmi faces filled with emotion, while Malu stood watching, eyes wide in surprise and terror.

Late that night, as I stirred in bed I heard Dad whisper to Mom, "Sunder was in the theater watching Alfred Hitchcock's suspense thriller, "Psycho." Doctors think he might have died of shock...it is a horror film.... suddenly a chair swings and there's a skeleton, you know."

He grunted and chuckled loud, while Mom also chuckled softly.

He continued with his suppressed whisper, "These young people! Why should they go to adult movies?"

Then after a few minutes, letting out a deep breath, "Why would he want to see such scary movies?"

The truth was out in a few days.

Sunder was declared dead due to his kidneys completely shutting down.

With his untimely death a few things happened. Our visits to Uncle Nara's became occasional and slowly tapered off to naught. The family in mourning found it hard to come to terms with their first child's abrupt exit from the world. They needed time and space to heal.

The fun times of family picnics were now some vague memories of the past.

Dad would bring fresh news now and then.

It was almost an annual event. Five of six kids in that family were sucked in by renal failure. Mysterious, clueless on what caused the disease that had dwelled in bodies of individuals we met almost every weekend. Among the kids disappearing in that household was my dear friend Malu. All memories of our play times were sealed in my brain's grey cells in a protective cage.

In those years, Uncle Nara slowly dug his grave, an ace marketing manager in the petroleum industry seemed too shocked with his inability to use his resources to change destiny of even one of his dying children. Aunt Laxmi held her last surviving kid close to her bosom as if challenging the demons, as any mother would protectively, guarding him from a powerful, destructive opponent.

In the dimmed lights of our household everyone spoke of these tragedies in undertones, lined with deep fear. All I knew was in kidney failure, people just died. I had to grow up to know more.

This happened in 1962 in Mumbai, India's premier city where doctors had only some basic information on renal failure. But there was lots of reservation in discussing the matter, explaining the treatment in as vague a manner as possible, exhibiting anxiety, lack of understanding on how to handle the patients, with limited scope of providing any positive solution. Limited knowledge and limited resources! Much has happened since then to renal world –in science through clinical work and people's understanding of the disease.

Nephrology, a study of renal disease became popular in first world countries like US and UK around 1960's. In ripple reaction organizations formed to do further research, support and make treatments available for this life-threatening disease. Not much has changed worldwide for this disease, as far as fear factor goes. Life seems unpredictable. Despite uncertainty hanging in the air, through research many solutions are found for people with disease to live good quality lives.

Vasundhara Raghavan

"CAN I BE OF ANY HELP, BROTHER?" – R. AND H.

When the World War II ended, a silence had settled world over, giving an opportunity to resume lives. Families with victims of war had to shed memories of their loved ones' and build their lives on hopes for better life in the future. They understood that time would heal their wounds. While parts of the world busied in serious business of developing the country or focusing on personal growth, some unsettled matters were bubbling in a hot pot.

One such lingering problem rocked Korea. Ruled by Japan from 1910 till end of World War II in 1945, who finally surrendered to American administrators who divided the Korean peninsula along the 38th parallel. This division meant that Republic of Korea was supported by the US with allied nations under the aegis of United Nations and the Democratic People's Republic of Korean was led by People's Republic of China, with military and material aid from USSR.

The constant tussle between the two powers, US and USSR with differing ideologies tore the fabric of Korea. North Korea had a single, planned development, while South Korea followed a free market, democratic economy. Living conditions were not normal and were subjected to lots of pressure from super powers.

The bubble burst on 25 June 1950.

Korean War broke out between the North and South Korea. US Military called able-bodied men to participate in the war at various military posts and services.

Among them were twin brothers, H and R. One received a posting in the Coast Guard, while the other was selected by the Army and was sent out at Germany. The brothers had left their father, brother V and a younger sister S, to join the services.

It was fortunate for them that they were far away from the intense war activity. They escaped the travails of living in high pressure war zone; they were not consumed by thirst for human blood, their night's sleep was peaceful and not interjected by hissing sounds of the bullet screeching by, they were not terrorized by oppression or starvation dealt to prisoners of war, they were also not subjected to unscrupulous massacre. Their time in service was far easy compared to many who were deeply involved in the war.

The war ended in July 1953.

The brothers planned their return homewards, with humaneness intact, holding love in their hearts. During the war their father had died and since they were motherless the family would now live with an aunt and uncle.

On the scheduled date H had arrived. The siblings and caregivers were concerned that R had not yet arrived.

Instead a shocking letter arrived from Marine Hospital, Chicago stating that they had been detained R, who was diagnosed with chronic kidney disease and was facing disorientation. The family was alarmed, *How could a normal, healthy young man be suddenly so disoriented? The letter had mentioned that toxins had accumulated in R's blood so that in manifested in a psychotic behavior.*

Suddenly, R's health and his survival posed greater uncertainty than days he spent serving in the war! R's death seemed most imminent and logical conclusion to the family.

Suddenly the tides changed. Concerned with R's condition, as the eldest sibling, V spoke to the doctor at US Public Health Service on what can be done to save R. The doctor recalled pioneering work being done in Peter Bent Brigham Hospital, Boston, Massachusettes where the first transplant was done in 1950 on a 44-year-old. Unfortunately the organ was rejected. (*Immunosuppressant therapy was non-existent at this time.*)

The doctor explained at length that in case of a tissue mismatch, the body considers the transplanted organ as a foreign object and rejects it. It dawned to the doctor that organ donation between twins will not face tissue compatibility issues. This triggered a new thought and H had elected to donate.

When they were admitted in the hospital for the transplant H had spent time recalling all that had been discussed and how things panned out in those early months.

'I want him back, safe and in normal health.

But is this worth experimenting?'

Meetings with the doctors, serious discussions involving his life and future, had tired him.

'Let me get it done and be in peace'.

He leaned back, closed his eyes.

'My first thought was to save R! I was keen and excited! But I also get so confused.'

H had felt a knot in the pit of his stomach. The thought that he was healthy and they would cut him open and take out one of his organs was alarming. Deep down there was some fear. The only surgery H ever had was an appendectomy, which he had not liked so much.

To H a kidney transplant was more in the realm of a science fiction. In such a tale he never dreamed he would be a participant. All through he had been in a dilemma; his mind had engaged itself in conflicting thoughts –to help his brother, but how would he go through such a major surgery!

Suddenly he had been disturbed by a faint knock that he chose to ignore.

Shifting to a more comfortable position, he focused on his thoughts.

During family discussions some worrying aspects came to the forefront. Clearly by now anxiety was for both the donor and recipient. Appropriately, the family raised the pertinent questions that the doctors fielded.

"What is the life expectancy of a person with one kidney?"

It was not difficult for the doctor to give a pat response, but it occurred to him that getting a third party assurance would break down the reservations.

The doctor approached insurance companies for accessing actuarial tables. After lengthy study the insurance companies made some unusual discovery and reported that there was no increased risk for living with one kidney. They talked of people born with a single kidney, which was found among one in a thousand.

Knock on the door had grown more insistent. His brows creased with slight irritation. *'This reflection is helping me clear my head... last few hours before dawn...and then...'*

But breathing deeply he had responded in a clear, loud voice.

"Please come in. The door is open."

The night nurse had entered the room the dark room, switched the light and with a bright smile, she had broken the heavy silence announcing,

11

"Check-up time!"

Noisily placing her nursing tray on the bedside table, she had popped the thermometer in his mouth, pulling out a note that she placed within his easy reach.

As she finished checking his vital signs, she had cleared her throat noisily. Looking straight into his eyes she said, "Your brother sent it for you".

Reaching out, H had picked up the note and read it slowly, once, twice.

"Get out of here and go home."

He had crushed the note in his right palm, his tight fist revealing pale, white knuckles. He was unhappy that his brother was still wavering, in spite of repeated assurances and topic discussed threadbare, concluded and sealed.

The nurse stood watching him, waiting for the next reaction. Scared and worried for being bearer of a letter sensitive to timing, made her wary.

'Did the contents disturb the young man?'

'Oh why, why did I take this risk? The doc will be furious!'

She stood silently wringing her hands, the left one and the right, all the time praying. The surgery was scheduled for early next morning. Hopefully she had not crushed the opportunity...so many people waited eagerly for this surgery.

'Now...have I endangered it?'

In the past few days she had watched the brothers battle out their emotions. She continued to chew her lower lip, as was her habit when facing uncomfortable moments.

Sitting upright on his chair, H collected his thoughts.

Picking up a note pad he began scribbling. Thoughts of his brother lying on the hard, uncomforting bed, pain keeping him restless, suddenly his expression softened. In that moment of calm, his mind got some clarity. With a lot more enthusiasm he wrote his brother a message that he would be proud of, for a long time to come.

"I am here and I am going to stay."

Folding the crisp note, H handed it to the nurse, saying,

"Madam, please give this note to my brother immediately.... before he retires."

The night was young. But high strung with emotion –one brother's mind swayed suggesting no surgery and the other emphatically knocked down his decision. In a glorious moment calm was established. World was put to rest as soon as decision was clamped.

Much after the nurse left, H sat thinking.

Another thought that crossed someone's mind. Without much ado, they placed it before the doctor.

"What are the chances of subsequent disease affecting the remaining kidney?"

Recognizing their mental turmoil, the doctors explained, "Most common types of renal disease affect both kidneys simultaneously. The most critical conditions affecting a solitary kidney are cancer and trauma, both fortunately rare".

These explanations brought great relief to the troubled family, who were looking for foolproof solutions. Now with full confidence they were ready excited to go ahead, do the surgery.

The matter rested thereafter with the doctors.

Huge responsibility was placed on doctors to plan and execute with precision.

Before attempting to open a healthy young man, the doctors wanted to do two things:

- A trial run

- A graft skin transplant from recipient to donor

As plans were afoot, for the first time they were stumped by an unusual situation, requiring revisiting their role.

Loyalties were now divided. Two people on the surgery table - one that needed it; one agreed to help.

Who would they bat for?

The obvious thing to do was to put all energies in cure of the patient who suffered from physical pain and traumatic episodes. After all weren't the doctors aware of his deteriorating condition and that any delay could cause a precious life?

Most tempting seemed to them was the aspect of testing out their theory of similar twins holding 100% tissue match! It could be a reason for long survival rates for kidney transplants!

The doctors agreed on their primary duty towards the patient.

But while calculations of nitty-gritty of the surgeries, their minds opened up and they deliberated on their roles in protecting the healthy man in a surgery where extensive surgical procedure would bring him no real benefit. In an unfortunate circumstance endangering his life to the extent any surgery does.

Troubled faces across the room suddenly showed a qualitative shift in their thinking. Surprisingly they unilaterally agreed the healthy person was someone to be watched out for.

Only after several levels of consultations within hospital, externally, including legal counsel the doctors decided. Yes they would do the surgery, with methodical planning, minute detailing and complete validation of results.

Though the surgery would be establishing a new procedure that would change world's perception on kidney disease and bring personal repute, it dimmed considering consequences of putting a healthy life in danger.

Suddenly all this reflection was tiring him. H looked at his watch and realised it was close to midnight. He should rest and be ready early for the surgery. He got up, stretched his body, and flexed his muscles. Now he felt relaxed. His brother's last message asking him to go home didn't detract him from doing what he had set out to do.

Feeling calmer he settled down for a restful sleep. In the morning there would be so much activity and excitement. The air was heavy with an element of suspense and curiosity. How successful will this 'experimental' surgery be?

The doctor knew this wasn't an experiment, but a natural transition to development of best medical practices taking surgery to its next level, from partial to confirmed success. Transplant without immunosuppressant needed 100% tissue match, so the twin brothers' case became a critical clinical study.

Even as the brother was being readied to donate his kidney, intensive study of getting the procedure right was taking place at the doctor's office. The doctor looked at minute details. Small mistakes –could mean balance could tip the other way. The doctor made copious notes, with a clinical report that had a blueprint for the surgery's procedure. Risky surgery needed meticulous planning to the dot.

Ingenious thinking was another highlight of the doctor's experimental surgery. To establish veracity of his theory that there was 100% match in the twins tissue, as an additional safeguard the doctor arranged for finger printing donor and recipient thumbs at the police station.

A newspaper reporter saw hospital staff making secret visits to the police station. Everything was being done in a hush! It raised a suspicion in Newspaper office. Suddenly this caused a stir.

"What was the strange business happening between the police station and hospital?" was the question in many minds.

News leaked out of *'unusual happenings'* at the Brigham Hospital.'

Slowly the story was out and the transplant became a sensational story.

There was a broadcast on a radio station with people tuned in to get every bit of information about the transplant. It became a day-to-day broadcast till the transplant was completed; this added pressure to perform successfully.

On the ethical part they maintained high levels of transparency in all discussions with the donor. In spite of it being their first possible chance for a successful transplant, the team placed all facts before the donor and his family, leaving them to make decisions without any remorse. These ingredients built in confidence in the donor and the public.

It is commendable that a detailed and systematic approach note was prepared and recorded introducing the clinical technique for a successful organ transplant. Minute details of the surgery were recorded which tells us the time taken for the each process; how the donor's kidney was transported in a wet, cold towel in a sterile basin. This establishes the fact that the surgeon had highly creative thinking, which when combined with proactive measures made this winning discovery.

With such a meticulous planning at the end of the day, a template for future transplants was ready.

Procedure: Identical -twin kidney transplant.
Date: December 23, 1954
Institution: Peter Bent Brigham Hospital, Boston, Massachusetts

The doctor masterminded a transplant that created a history of the first long surviving kidney transplant without immunosuppressant medications. The tissue of monozygotic (identical) twins being compatible was used as to understand how far this surgery could bring relief.

The story is extraordinary at many levels

- H offering his kidney when there was no known success rates for long-term successful organ donations. His offer was self-motivated and purely an act of love
- R survived the transplant and lived for 8 years thereafter
- Their parents were not alive to see this great feat by the operating surgeon nor the love and bonding their children shared
- It became the winning experiment creating history in the field of nephrology. It was *'this magical first transplant'* that paved the way for organ transplants in other parts of the world. Kidney patients saw opportunity for relief and to lead normal lives!

H was driven by a sense of duty, without batting an eyelid he agreed to donate his kidney. It was in his words *"in the realm a science fiction"*. The doctor was honored with a Nobel Prize for medicine in 1990.

Source: *Surgery of the Soul, by Dr Joseph Murray*

Story dramatized to showcase the spectacular case.

EARLY LESSONS – SUSAN AND RICHARD

She stood near the pot and saw her urine had small spots of blood. Eyes wide with wonder she inspected the toilet seat. It had no trace of blood. But she was confused. What was this? Twisting the frock at the hem, she stepped out of the toilet nervously. But that was momentary. No sooner she heard her brother shout out to her, she tossed her head and fear away, "Susan, come soon. It's now your turn to give the den."

Susan ran back excited. She wanted to catch the thief soon. Last time her chance was squashed. What a shame!

Next day, when she peeked into the pot, again it was the same. Urine had small specs of blood. Now her fear resurfaced.

She walked out quietly and went straight to her mother.

"Mother...Mother..."

She stopped... not clear on what to say next.

"What's it Susan? Be quick, I'm busy. Need to finish this fast and get ready for dinner." She was busy wrapping up her unfinished deskwork. Seeing Millie silent, hesitant, looking a bit confused her mother got anxious.

Fortunately Susan was extremely smart. Realising it was best to show proof-of-evidence she took her Mother's hand and walked her to the toilet.

What her Mother saw drew breath out of her! Settling six-year-old Millie on a high stool she asked some questions. Susan could answer all but one –what had happened to her?

The next day they took the road to the nearest clinic. After several days of physical examinations and unique tests one doctor detected something far more serious than Millie could comprehend let alone, handle. What the doctor said was a shocking revelation even for the parents.

"I think Susan has some kind of kidney disease. It is known as Bright's disease or *Gluomeronephtitis*... At some point her kidneys may shut down completely. Till then we need to take extreme care. Hopefully it will happen progressively."

Susan's Mom realized the magnanimity of the challenge that lay ahead.

'This will be huge, very huge. How would I save my daughter from this insurmountable disease?'

Those were times when little was known of the disease. But with some guidance from the physician the mother established basic precautions of living with the disease.

This early introduction into safe measures proved useful as Susan managed to hold her life together, for nearly four decades. Was it a streak of courage that held her life together? Was she prepared for what was round the bend and know the next great changer in her life? Was it pure luck, is anyone's guess.

Everything is merely speculative.

Susan married George, an engineer, who being highly educated had a better understanding of the seriousness of the disease. This union possibly made great impact on how her disease was managed.

George and Susan were overjoyed with the birth of their son, Frank and his younger brother Richard in 1952 and1956. Even as their lives filled with joy, tides of pain lashed the walls of their strong fortress, threatening to shatter it.

At an early age, traces of blood were found in Brian's urine.

Susan picked up the cue and knew where his kidney was heading. Understanding basic issues, managing situations and wearing brave smiles the couple encouraged and educated Richard on what he should expect.

In a few years Susan developed high blood pressure, which culminated in nephrosclerosis [hardening of the nephrons] as revealed by a kidney biopsy.

In 1983, at 27 years, an episode of gout showed Richard the dark face of the disease. Doctors confirmed it was *Gluomeronephtitis*.

The next eight years witnessed a slow but steady decline in Richard's kidney function. As if cocooned into a world of his own he slogged to graduate with a doctorate in Philosophy. He became an Assistant Professor. His family had an addition at this stage, as his wife gave him a baby. Richard's life seemed blissful. In the darkness of a closet, between piles of linen, the disease lay trapped. To let it lie there, Richard remained on low protein, low salt diet, which helped delaying the kidney failure by a few years. But the disease sneered at him, kept him constantly tired and was slowly growing to overwhelm him.

In 1986 Susan's kidney showed signs of shutting down. She started dialysis a year later.

It seemed the mother-son duo went through stages of disease one leading, the other following at arm's length. There was show of courage and forbearance, masking deep emotional turbulence that lay possibly below the surface.

Year 1990 saw both mother and son at the dialysis center.

Mom and Son matching dates for disease, dialysis and transplant

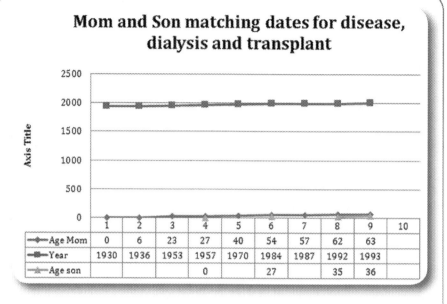

Mom and Son matching dates for disease, dialysis and transplant

	1	2	3	4	5	6	7	8	9	10
Age Mom	0	6	23	27	40	54	57	62	63	
Year	1930	1936	1953	1957	1970	1984	1987	1992	1993	
Age son				0		27		35	36	

Susan born 1929; 1935 detected; 1952 first son; 1956 Richard's birth; 1964 high BP; 1986 confirmed; 1987-1992 dialysis; 1992 Transplant (Tx) Richard born 1957; 1983 confirmed; 1990 dialysis; 1992 Tx

George had a formidable task. Saving lives of two very dear people, his wife and son —one who had seen different facets of the life-threatening disease and the other carried hope in his eager, young eyes.

It meant being mentally alert, enough to maintain stability and find latest medical advancements. Susan's foray into dialysis began with CAPD to give a better life-style. But she experienced seven episodes of peritonitis. Under duress she was compelled to change to hemodialysis —which meant greater diet restrictions and a greatly diminished lifestyle. Strict on diet, low on fluid intake, high doses of EPO yet she remained tired, fought sleeplessness, developed cough and breathing problems caused by fluid buildup. High blood pressure was a major stumbling block, where listing for organ transplant was concerned. Many prominent medical centers evaluated and rejected her candidature.

George had to find that one missing link that would nail their problems and bring long lasting relief for the whole family.

George's unequivocal support through Susan's toughest periods can only be imagined. Watching her in pain, helping in lifting CAPD bags, or look out when the cycler machine beeped. One could detect sad and happy periods and wonder how his waking hours was singularly directed towards securing the lives of two members facing grave health conditions.

In Susan's eyes, pain was visible as well as disappointment to see her son stretched on the clinic bed, being dialyzed with needles pricking him. No matter that Richard consoled her on many occasions. But she knew well, what those tubes did in the process of bringing out blood to clean it, while keeping the person strapped. She knew well, the nauseous feeling, the cramps and feeling of lowness.

The person, who bore it silently watching from the distance and mulling over it all, was Richard's elder brother Frank. As a son and brother, all through his growing years he had witnessed, how the disease had troubled his mother and in later years, his kid brother Richard joined her brigade. How it impacted Frank's life was never a subject of discussion. But it is true that every family member gets deeply affected by the strains of the disease.

In a unique manner, Frank chose to play monitor, kept a tab on the disease's progression and at an appropriate moment, he encouraged Susan to undergo an evaluation for transplant. But her uncontrolled blood pressure became an impediment and the centers discouraged her, explaining how it could prove a disastrous for her.

Richard managed his disease responsibly bringing some sense of relief to his parents.

If one peeked through their windows one would notice a busy household. But if one is intent, it will not escape their notice that most activity surrounded the patients and their medical treatments. Stepping back, the observer will leave a deep breath and marvel at the family's determination to learn new ways to understand and accept their life's challenges.

Frank was considered as a probable donor for Richard, but initial tests showed there was no match of blood group. Providence showed George's kidney matched with Richard and then with some persuasion, the center agreed to Frank donating to Susan as they had the same blood type. Miraculously doctors were willing to go ahead with Susan's transplant!

30th July1992 Richard had his transplant and his mother had hers two months later.

The fear of age being criteria for rejecting the surgery drove Susan (62 years) and George (64 years) to work towards getting physically fit. They paved the way for changing opportunities into destinies.

As he looks back, Richard appreciates the kind of change the disease made to his life. The pain and suffering being part and parcel of the disease, groomed him to be a far greater human being, with compassion and understanding of human lives. He truly values the gift of the disease.

The underlying success mantra:

Factors that contributed to this family's achievement:

- *Opening doors to knowledge. Awareness of the issues related to kidney failure*
- *Emotional bondage and appreciation of the intensity of pain of two members*
- *Embarking on the road to kidney transplant single mindedly*
- *No compulsions, no differing views*

- *Clear on the single purpose of life*
- *Dedicated commitment among family members*

After the transplant the family shared their experiences on transplants and explained how it had enriched their lives. Each member of the family approached the topic from their perceptive. Their aim was on encouraging living donor related transplants.

Story based on information supplied by George with whom the author was in touch till 2013. Family had a website that provided updates. Susan's death unrelated to the kidney disease was shared at some point. The website has recently been disabled. Respecting privacy names have been changed.

COURAGE GROWS WITH
COMPLICATIONS – KELLY FRANCIS

"Mom, I will be late tonight... its girl's night out," Kelly said nonchalantly.

It took a moment longer for her to realize that she was being abrupt and rude. Biting her lower lip, she realized how deeply her attitude would hurt her mother. Wiping clean every trace of indifference in her behavior, she flashed a bright smile, as she walked up to her mother, hugged her briefly and spoke in an excited voice, "Mom, I forgot to mention it earlier. 'Eleanor' has a wonderful late evening sale, to launch their new season collection. It's tomorrow at 7pm... Shall we do dinner at 'The Wok' and shop at the store? I haven't been there in a while."

"Ah, that will be wonderful, Kelly. I was meaning to do some clothes shopping before going on my holiday."

"So it's a plan, Mom. Let's do it. I will ask Myra to book a table at 6pm...."

Picking up her car keys, she looked back and added, "...will be back latest by eleven. Goodnight Mom."

Kelly walked out swiftly. She was late by a few minutes for the blind date. Lisa and Henry would join them later at the pub.

Her mother was glad that they planned a dinner for the next day. But after a while she went back to her evening's muse and became thoughtful. Seeing Kelly young, beautiful and so full of life always made her happy.

But since past few months she had noticed something...she was unable to understand what had happened, but all the same. In quieter moments, she consoled herself that Kelly was no longer a kid and as a young woman these changes were part of emerging as a young lady holding a top position in the fashion world.

No matter what, she felt some discomfort about which she couldn't share with anyone.

At times she blamed Kelly for her great weakness to partying heavily. Weekends were completely spent with friends, with little rest before start of another long week. Her work as head of sales and marketing at "Elitist" kept her busy on week days, where she worked hard for long hours and returned home late, exhausted.

Kelly loved her work.

What a wonderful work environment! Chic and modern – most happening place for young go-getters! People were drawn here due to creative layouts, exciting offers and wonderful selection of fabric, textures and accessories. Other than organizing the store displays and promotions her knowledge of designs made her a resource for sourcing products across many suppliers.

Kelly was a decision maker and her skills were amply recognized and rewarded by the employers. Her dedication and involvement made her indispensable. Work was very stressful but she managed it well.

There was one thing that she regretted.

With such heavy schedules she was unable to find enough time to spend with her mother. She hated it that her being busy extracurricular activities meant at times neglecting her mom, her best friend and mentor. She never forgot how hard her Mom had worked, made many personal sacrifices to see Kelly got educated and graduated too.

Her personal ambitions and need for a life-partner had fueled many pre-occupations in her life. Kelly dreamed of opening her own store under a joint venture with a famed designer. Life was on a high, and she wanted to accomplish a lot.

Next morning even as her mind was racing, one hand on the car's steering wheel and the other busy getting her phone active Kelly called her Mom, "Hey, Mom...so you remember our evening's program?"

"Hey Kelly, yes I'm looking forward to it. I will drive over at quarter to six."

"See you Mom!"

It was a hectic working day for Kelly as they had annual stocktaking.

Before mid-day surprisingly she was exhausted. By noon her weakness persisted and it looked like she would collapse. With great difficulty she picked up her cell-phone and dialed the last number.

"Something very funny has happened! Since morning I am feeling very low and exhausted. I am unable to do any work!"

"Kelly, it may be your partying late last night!"

She whispered back, "Mom...! Too weak to fight with you...there's no energy left."

"Kelly...I think you need to get yourself checked. Go to "Good Samaritan" and see a doctor. I will join you there."

Taking cue from her mother's advice she left work, excusing herself for a few hours. The hospital was just two blocks away. She parked her car with great difficulty and was almost swooning when she entered the lobby. Though extremely tired she managed to fill the personal information and insurance details.

Her mother walked in saying, "There you are! Oh, Kelly you do look pale."

Just then the assistant called, "Kelly Francis!"

The doctor was friendly and asked many questions. Kelly answered politely though she wanted to just get some quick fix to her health problem and run back to the store.

The doctor put her through several tests. They met again after a couple of hours. Studying the reports the doctor seemed disappointed when he said, "I am sorry, but things do not seem good as far as your health is concerned. Blood pressure is very high. The blood test shows high levels of creatinine. It looks like you are heading towards a kidney failure."

"Doctor, what is creatinine, I mean what does it do?" Kelly asked vaguely as this word didn't ring any bell.

"Ms Kelly, creatinine is a chemical waste product in the blood that goes to the kidney so that it gets rid off through the urine. Levels of creatinine indicate how well the kidney is functioning. So one may say your kidney functions are impaired."

Twenty-year-old Kelly was too stunned to utter a word.

As soon as she collected her thoughts she asked the one question that bothered her, "How did it happen? What triggered it?"

The doctor nodded, "You need to do more tests. Get a sonography and a chest x-ray. Then we will get a clear picture."

The initial tests were enough to create panic in mother and daughter. Kelly was distraught and had no idea how to manage her health. Gathering all the courage to find solutions, Kelly's mother started discussing with the doctor on the kind of treatments that Kelly would need to keep fine. Even after a battery of tests, the doctor could not draw any conclusion on what had caused the kidney failure. But it was confirmed that she would be starting dialysis very soon.

With her mother by her side, Kelly took stock of the situation.

She studied the various options for dialysis and decided to go for peritoneal dialysis (PD). With PD she would be able to manage life with reasonable comfort.

Gradually Kelly's life changed. Gone were days of hectic partying. Her health care occupied most of her time. To begin with her hemoglobin was low. To treat her anemic condition she was given erythropoietin (anemia correcting hormone) at regular intervals.

But as one problem got resolved, another cropped up. They were like unwelcome guests knocking at her door now and then.

Several weeks later she noticed change in her skin. It became so itchy that it grew rough and red. Applying calamine lotions gave her only temporary relief.

Her blood test helped her to catch the culprit. Phosphorus was rising rapidly. Managing with food charts given by the doctor on foods with high phosphorus kept her worried but it was very difficult to put good information to use. Finally she approached a dietician explaining her problem.

"From your blood report it is clear that higher levels of phosphorus is creating the problem. This means you need to restrict intake of food high in phosphorus. Without limiting food with phosphorus content, you'll land yourself in a serious problem. Lowering phosphorus will stop this itchiness. Try some of these," she said handing her some leaflets.

Drawing her into conversation, the dietician asked her to share her diet.

Though Kelly was concerned with her health and the severe itching, when the dietician probed on her food habits she was hesitant. Gradually the cat was out of the bag. Kelly loved her comfort food of pizzas and cola drinks. The dietician suggested option of low fat cream cheese as a substitute for cheese to be eaten on toast with vegetables like lettuce, bell peppers, onion and cucumber, suggested limiting consumption of such fast foods by adopting a more healthy diet. She talked of whole grains and fresh vegetables and suggested snacks like carrot sticks, apple or a simple cucumber sandwich to satisfy hunger and also improve her health. She concluded, "A little management of diet through restriction of foods, such as dairy products, will help in curbing the rampantly growing phosphorus. Additionally your doctor will prescribe phosphorus binders that will bind it in your intestines. It will help you."

Much as she tried Kelly's phosphorus remained unrestrained. It was tough for her to choose alternative food to reduce her phosphorus levels.

Problems escalated for Kelly when new issues developed. Her blood test gave another alert –Elevated parathyroid hormone. This spelt problem exposing her to associated complications that could end in bone disease, skin problem, anemia and cardiovascular disease.

She was advised medical therapy for lowering levels of parathyroid hormones.

It was mid morning on a summer day, Kelly had just left the doctor's clinic and was feeling cold. She decided to go to the cafeteria for a hot drink and spend time trying to understand where her life was heading. She sat at a corner table in the hospital's cafeteria, huddled to keep warm, feeling burdened with pressures of health and life in general. At this hour there was a thin crowd. Sipping into her coffee she let her thoughts go back to a past, that she had forsaken a long while back when caught by the fangs of chronic kidney disease. "I was always an author of my destiny till now. Now life is slipping away so fast. So many minor issues turning to major health problems are coming up. Will I ever get back control of my health?"

Tears were threatening to flow as she saw it as a losing game, "This is something beyond my capacity to understand and so huge! How will I retrace steps and get my stability back. I had built her life from naught; was the sole provider for Mom and me. What will happen to us?"

The coffee did little to give her any peace. Collecting her bag she left the hospital resigning to destiny to direct and lead her.

Very soon it became obvious that there was no way she could get a handle on the vagrant blood levels, in spite of efforts and slowly she was drawn into major surgeries.

She developed hyperparathyroidism, a tumor developed in the parathyroid glands, which showed her calcium levels had peaked. To bring some sense to her health, which was taking many plunges and set her free it was necessary to remove 3½ of 4 parathyroid glands. With several weeks of calcium and vitamin D therapy, her condition stabilized and blood levels showed improvement in phosphorus levels.

There's no boundary for pain and sufferance in kidney patients. Kelly was put to her next test. Years of peritoneal dialysis wore her peritoneum lining thin. It came to her notice when she started experiencing night sweats, fatigue, abdominal pain, and intermittent fevers.

The nephrologist suspected abdominal tuberculosis. He arranged peritoneoscopy (a procedure to look into her abdomen to evaluate peritoneal membrane's condition). Under the powerful machine, the membrane looked abnormal. A biopsy of an abdominal gland showed tuberculosis (TB) as positive.

Treatment for TB was commenced, but a serious liver complication developed due to the TB drug. She was put on a long hospital stay to make full recovery possible. The nephrologist permitted alternative medication to her TB regimen, to accelerate recovery.

Though she was very comfortable with PD, her membrane was unable to survive this onslaught, so she switched to hemodialysis (HD).

Kelly braved through various complications that rocked the boat of her life and stayed cheerful. With eyes filled with hope and dreams, she awaits now for a kidney for transplant.

> In kidney disease diet plays a great role. Limiting foods high in phosphorus could have helped Kelly. Making right food choices is a science by itself. It needs lots of dedicated attention to get it right. In the case of excess phosphorus, which cannot be removed by a diseased kidney, chances of it affecting the bones and parathyroid glands makes it an important mineral to watch out so a slow performing kidney is not burdened. Eating *forbidden food* as one may refer to chocolates, cheese, meat and other phosphorus food, must be seriously considered to avoid adverse health conditions.

> Judging people who failed to manage their blood levels is easy from the comfort of our armchairs, but bringing the balance in reality is very tough. One has to deal with sodium, phosphorus, potassium, blood sugar and protein. In specific cases minerals like magnesium could also be an issue. With kidney getting diseased, unable to perform its function completely, the balance can tip very fast. Health is unpredictable. But it's important to understand that managing a dialysis diet is a huge challenge for everyone.

I FOUND PEACE THROUGH
ACCEPTANCE – TOM CARTER

Tom Carter stood watching Susan leave with her baby.

"Ha! Now Mary and I can spend a quiet evening...maybe a chilled beer...some baked pita chips, olives and salsa!" were thoughts racing through his brain as he smacked his dry lips, and sank comfortably into his black leather study chair.

"Need to complete this assignment quickly..." he reminded himself as he hooked his reading spectacles on his nose bridge and opened the document on his mac.

Suddenly it seemed as if words were just tumbling out.

'Now I can do without such interruptions! The spectacle needs cleaning!' Reaching for a tissue he worked aggressively, irritation evident on his otherwise calm face.

The spectacles fixed but without any improved result.

"What's wrong with me? Why is my vision suddenly blurred?"

With a growing fear he realized that something was seriously wrong with his eyes. Every time he attempted to read, it was a similar experience. Sinking back in his chair, he grappled trying to recover balance.

But forces unknown to him squashed his feeble, panic attempts taking his body into a depth of shrouded darkness.

It was well after seven when Mary entered his study.

"Tom! Why in heavens are you working in darkness?"

Normally, he would let out a loud chuckle at being disturbed or being reprimanded. But she was met with silence. She groped for the switch and finding it turned on his table lamp. Under its brilliance, she saw Tom was slumped, shoulders hunched.

She rushed across to Tom, anxiously shaking him to bring him out of his stupor. But he was unnerved. Her heart was in a state of flutter, as she dialed #911.

Within minutes the emergency services arrived. Quickly reacting to the situation the technician checked Tom's vital signs. Quietly attaching the oxygen mask, programming the machine they moved him into the waiting ambulance, shutting the door on Mary, her pale face still in a state of shock. As the ambulance left the porch, she got into the car to drive to the hospital.

By the time Tom arrived at the facility he was partially revived. At the admission, the nurse approached Mary with a list of questions.

"Hi, I am Sarah...nurse in attendance to..."

Mary was very anxious but managed a weak smile. Wringing her palms she interrupted with her own questions, "How is my husband? What went wrong? He was fine some hours back and...I did not look up on him as he was busy completing a project..."

"Please calm down Mrs..."

"Call me Mary Carter, please...how is Tom?"

"Mr Carter will be fine in sometime. He was weak and exhausted. We decided to give him some rest. In the meanwhile I will need some basic information..."

Sarah noted basic information on her data collection sheet.

'Age-51 years'

Social Security...

Mary was tired, worried.

The nurse was a warm and understanding person. She was chirpy and quickly comforted Mary, handing her a mug with a freshly brewed coffee, "Mrs Carter you just need to relax a bit."

A few minutes later, returning with initial reports she shared the results of the test, "His blood count is very low. That shows how anemic he is! We will be doing other tests and will bring you up to speed."

It was sometime later when the nurse took Mary to meet Tom. Patting the leather couch she added, "I think you will like to stay with him. I will stop by later with a pillow and some sheets."

Turning back she suggested, "The cafeteria will close soon. If you want to get a snack...I can watch over Mr Carter!"

Mary responded with a tight smile, "I'm fine."

She watched Tom's steady breath and gradually got into a more comfortable position. "I need to keep alert. How did it happen...I was absolutely unaware that he had collapsed?"

Over the next few days X-rays, blood and 24-hour urine revealed many new areas for worry.

Tests showed presence of serum protein. That confirmed reason for Tom's anemic condition!

It took a protein electrophoresis to draw a conclusion that it was an abnormality in plasma cell formation, unusually high white cells that were growing fast in numbers. The bone-marrow biopsy nailed it as blood cancer known as 'multiple myeloma.'

But the worst was yet to come.

Susan was visiting with her husband. While they were busy with the Baby, nurse Sarah entered with fresh update on Tom's health. "I'm afraid it's bad news... your kidneys are severely damaged. You need immediate dialysis to sustain life."

Promising to come by in sometime she left Tom in a state of shock and devastated.

Opening his heart to Mary he said, "It's almost like she has been awarded me a death sentence! Oh...now what! It's just so sudden." Eyes brimming with unshed tears, shaking his head he said dejectedly, "No idea my life was heading this way... end is so near!"

Mary held his hands and looking into his eyes she said reassuringly, "Tom, there are treatments available. Let's get them started... there's hope for survival. Please let's explore..."

Then in her usual firm tone she added, "...and most certainly don't give up."

Talking to Mary changed Tom's mood magically.

Deep concern was visible in her transparent blue eyes; her grasp was warm, showing how much Tom meant to her. Her love and support brought a new confidence and sense of belonging in the middle-aged man, whose wrinkled eyes now carried love of life.

Susan got briefed of Tom's diagnosis. Her eyes were moist but with an effort she winked at her Dad, smiling warmly, encouragingly. Mary, Susan and her husband watched Tom with abated breath hoping he would decide quickly. There was worry that such a complicated disease would destroy him.

Tom said a silent prayer and thought "I still have enough life in me..."

The next morning Tom informed the doctor of his decision. Immediately he began his treatments. Special chemotherapy was scheduled and he would start dialysis thrice a week, along with blood transfusions. Depending upon his body's response to therapy further course would be determined.

Tom hated dialysis and believed it was an error of judgment. He questioned the doctors closely wonderingly, and being an optimist he was sure one day his normal kidney function would return.

Tom's hemoglobin levels improved, and myeloma stabilized with treatment and erythropoietin. If only he would not need dialysis!

> If one could avoid dialysis many people would be living happily free of such hassle. Dialysis as a treatment is universally disliked. In 1943 Dr Willem Kolff constructed the first dialysis machine. His mission for change began when he had helplessly watched a young man die due to kidney failure. Stumbling upon an article published in 2013 on hemodialysis for animals, he was encouraged to explore further. Today dialysis is the first stage of treatment for people all over the world as it effectively removes toxins accumulated in the blood stream due to poor kidney functions. One can't imagine how people with kidney disease could have survived without some kind of dialysis being available.

> Though Tom resented it very soon he realized how dialysis was keeping him comfortable. Gradually he learnt to carry on life with this regime.

> Tom had certainly no way to control any of it. Myeloma and dialysis came accidently into his life. Mary watches him manage his life. She is grateful that his life was saved. The call for 911 was indeed made at the right time.

MANAGE OR YOU WILL WANE
– ABBOTT STANLEY

Abbott Stanley lay uneasily on his bed, eyes searching the ceiling for inspiration. It was clinic day. His hands crept downwards reaching to where his torso ended. Beyond that he had nothing more to touch. His lips twitched into a smile, tinged with pain and sarcasm. The extent his body was abused by the illness was unbelievable. In some time he would be assisted to dress and he would leave.

On many a morning his thoughts would race back to the past, reliving those priceless moments. Every ounce of energy that flowed now came from memories of the distant past that continued to bring him joy. His eyes would grow luminous with some sparks of life and his lips would spread into a smile... just for a few minutes he would give his deep hurt a miss.

My childhood dreams and ambitions of becoming a surgeon, operating on people and saving their lives....it happened just as I wanted...how glad I am for this chance... many challenges came my way ...I dared to face them ...as other aspirants did ...Finally that wonderful moment-as I walked down the white hospital corridor... the matron and duty nurse...called out.....”Welcome Doctor” and congratulations poured from all quarters....the most wonderful party later that evening...

I was standing near the table laid with bouquets, dainty cup cakes, and a big spread of appetizers...someone unscrewed a bottle of sparkling French champagne... Dad and Mom were standing at a distance...as Deputy raised the toast Dad and Mom found a way to come close to me...I turned to look at Dad...he wore a large smile and raised the toast...I saw Mom’s eyes brim with tears of joy... how proud they felt... I felt good, real good... I knew that my ambitious streak, competitiveness, dedication and hard work had helped.

My many years as a vascular surgeon performing complicated surgeries... it was always satisfying to see someone cured and return home to their family...

And Ah.... those lectures I imparted...how much I loved it! Freshman, medical graduate students and trainees too...they gained on critical aspects of surgery... showing my patients value of personal targets in health care... publishing scientific papers...my own contributions to the medical world. I had achieved it all.... Meeting my goals, delivering to my greatest potential... life had been smooth sailing... it brought in loads of appreciation, feeling of great achievement, glorious period that it was! Best moments wrapped together...

Lots of work...lots of surgeries...many conferences...new breakthroughs...no time to sit and enjoy the moment...it was all lovely moments piled one on another...hope I had taken a short holiday and spent time with Dad and Mom...how often she called and asked me to come and I called last minute to cancel my visit...I made them sad...they knew I was busy...but if only I had managed to do that...maybe things would be different.

And then... that day...a warm, sunny day...but yet, I was shivering... a dark, shrouded stranger met me as I left the clinic... I walked and he followed at a distance. At home when I took my first sip of single malt...there was a knock on the door...I opened the door, bowing he introduced himself, "I am diabetes," he said, "and I am here to stay with you..."

Abbott lay in his bed; the smile faded and replaced by a distant look, eyes dark, glistening with pain and emotion. He recalled his reactions at that time.

How vehemently I had refused to entertain the visitor - "it cannot be me", is what I said repeatedly. I am a learned surgeon, I would have known everything about health matters, is what my mind said...later when it got confirmed how much it hurt to know that I had been caught unaware. I had to be reminded...diabetes is a silent and heartless disease.

Heartless, because it changed my lifestyle! It restricted me from eating my favorite dishes... how very heartless.

When my patients learnt to manage their illnesses and handle post-operative care as advised...it was so satisfying... sometimes I felt remorse when the case was hopeless.

But in my own case...how did I not do it right? Truth hurts, and it hurts so badly!

My entry into rough weathers with diabetes was a different experience...as reality sank in I stepped into patient shoes with the gambit of periodic checking blood sugar levels and giving insulin shots while maintaining a busy career as a surgeon.

But it was late, very late when I knew my condition. I did my best, but slowly every door seemed to shut on me.

I was devastated as diabetes played havoc with my body...my diminished eye sight affected my surgical skills...with peripheral circulatory my nervous system got badly affected and the feeling in my lower extremities was extremely reduced...I felt as if I was walking on cotton wool.

I had difficulty in maintaining an erect posture over long periods.... my autonomic system had been severely damaged...poor blood circulation led to my losing one leg.... then the other...But... I learnt to manage with the prosthetic limb and later, on the wheelchair!

Imagine... from a very active surgeon I became a wheelchair bound patient. Only my extensive reading brought me peace... being sociable also helped. Unfortunately, my kidneys failed and I needed dialysis. Hemodialysis, dietary restrictions, medications to control anemia, phosphorous, hemoglobin, blood pressure and diabetes became part and parcel of my life.

I wish some complications had been arrested. I would be happier today for those chances.

Then with a smile brightening his face he thought, *But how can I forget those wonderful trips to meet friends...yes they were good, going out of Oregon was my real escape... those were like adventures...away from this life...strapped on the bed or wheelchair.*

Today was different. Abbott spent more time analyzing his life, than before. He became more questioning.

How did I manage all these debacles in life? Why did I let myself land from one stage to another? Is it possible that at times I was not compliant with diet and medication? I fooled myself into thinking that I did it well.

As problems kept piling on ...I saw reason to go with the tide ... dread of dialysis evoked fear and possibility of a bleak end...but I stayed composed... To best of my ability I kept pace with changes happening at each stage.

His eyes moist with tears but the insides hurt treacherously, the unbearable pain shook his body all over and he showed little struggle to maintain himself.... no more of this...his eyes were closed...his emotions took over and submerged him under pressure of wretchedness...Soon time to retrospect was past... slowly his body collapsed... and he took his last breadth...now totally in peace.

Everyone remembered Abbott for his charming manners, determination, and sense of humor. Most importantly people appreciated his forbearance. In him they saw acceptance of the disease and fighting every stage of illness as the attitude to be emulated by patients arriving at this stage in illness. In admiration the nephrologists, nurses, dietitian, social workers and other professionals offered him encouragement and supported emotionally.

The stages of illness, the pain, fear and sorrow associated is beyond everyone's capacity to endure.

But one can wonder what went through his mind as he went through helplessly letting go of some part of him. Did he accuse himself for being so naïve not to see it coming? Early detection, timely action could have stalled progression, after all he advised his patients to be medically compliant. But now, what? Loosing body parts, fighting for survival, letting destiny shape his life when his fight failed, was it just too many things to handle?

This could happen to you or me if we do not understand value of curbing desire to splurge and land ourselves into health crisis. After all isn't it all about living in moderation? Eat well, live right, see beyond just plain life and achieve much more. Living life to the fullest need not be in total abandon.

The story of this surgeon however, showed something very remarkable.

In death society continued to respect him and recognize his surgical talents. A man who lost all else carried his reputation untarnished shows a special place he held in a world that did not judge him as being a bad patient. His work determined his true position.

Thankfully he was not an object of pity. In public mind he remained a man of great stature.

It's very common for people to be very pre-occupied with daily activities. Chance of ignoring health is easy, as one tends to take health for granted. In this case the doctor was so engrossed in caring for patients and he placed greater credence to their recovery. He never paused to wonder, "Am

I eating properly? Am I feeling thirsty often?" He put other lives as priority. Wake-up call came too late. Thereafter struggling to catch up missed alert signs only shows lost opportunity and fills a bag full of regrets. Abbot had people who respected him. But for a common man such a health complication can draw flak from society. World admires winners and ignores losers.

In the game of dice the probability of it falling face up with all six dots at every throw is improbable. Far fetched even for very deft sportsperson. The same is also true for human beings, not everyone can be a winner. Life may become a dark road that could lighten up when an extraordinary power magically transforms the darkness. Not all lives get chosen for such miraculous escapade. Respect for humanity irrespective of face up or down must be our endeavor leaving judgment to those empowered.

As we crawl in the twilight of our life everything will become crystal clear. We will no longer think of the right or wrong, black or white but will see it gray in its simplest form. As truly there's never a winner or loser; it was the statistical probability of a dice falling face up that had sealed the fate.

PEOPLE TALK—CONTROL
PHOSPHORUS – LUCY DREW

The middle aged lady sat straight back in a chair by the window, her trembling fingers rolled the rosary beads, as her lips murmured soundlessly, in worship. Her face was taut, eyes glistened with unshed tears. Her mind was busy with thoughts.

It was about Lucy, her daughter, her child. She worried about Lucy all the time. How can she ever forget what a gruesome life Lucy had lived not too long back!

The mother knew tomorrow's sunrise would bring joyful showers of flowers, champagne glasses would be raised to toast for Lucy and Robert by many family members and close friends. Many people who would bless Lucy, as she was much loved.

She walked to the dresser to dab some face powder and taint her tired eyes that lacked luster due to sleepless nights. "I should be happy, relaxed now. Why is my forehead wrinkled with worry? Why should I remember those by gone days when my most loved child Lucy, face near death situation? Why cannot I love her and laugh with her today?" the mother questioned her silly behavior! But what could she do! Those memories were still so strong and fresh.

She remembered that day very well. It came back in a flash.

It was the great countdown to the millennium. World was maneuvered to believe even the sun's glory would change. Some imaginary wheels will move them physically from 20th to the 21st century. Euphoria and excitement drove party planning on new concepts world over. It was simply not like another year-end party.

The Canton household always partied in style. They readied to celebrate the turn of the century with great fanfare. So adept they were in doing things with aplomb, the barbeque aflame, grilling thick, juicy steaks, the bar opened with glasses waiting to be filled, liquor bottles stacked neatly, chilled wine and beer left refrigerated, and large platters of grilled vegetables, small chicken tarts, burgers and chips, cheese and crackers all plated to please different palates.

Plan was to warm the floor till late night with alcohol freely flowing, till everyone was ready to drop dead. Speculations were rift on year 2000 breaking all barriers, economically and socially. World would be one great place to exist.

Guests came in, leaving a trail of mixed fragrance. But Lucy who was fully keyed on the celebration was showing signs of fatigue, and discomfort, the kind she couldn't understand. But she decided to remain cheerful and let her hair down, with the blaring music. A few hours later, much before midnight, she felt she would collapse. She retired quietly to her room. She would rest a little.

It was the morning rays of the sun that stirred her out of her deep slumber. But Lucy was still feeling odd, uneasy.

The parents were concerned that Lucy had retired early the night before while guests were asking for her. Seeing her under the weather, the mother rushed her to the clinic. The senior doctor began tests, starting with the blood pressure.

"I find your high blood pressure is high. We need to do some more tests. In the meantime you must start some medicines to control your blood pressure." The doctor started a battery of tests. It revealed chronic kidney disease caused by hypertension. Lucy was put on health alert. Diet and medications were advised, along with dialysis. In sync with her attitude and lifestyle, she opted for peritoneal dialysis. She enjoyed life, within restrictions placed by her health condition.

But something happened to bring her joy to an abrupt end. Peritonitis inflamed her abdominal wall and she was hospitalised. Under expert care, she recovered after an antibiotic therapy. Health restored, she bounced back to life's routine with her PD. This was a 'less stressed about health' phase.

As she watched with love and concern, the mother's stomach curled with tension. When Lucy was out off the routine hospital visits she quickly settled down back to PD. She seemed happy.

What will happen to Lucy? Was her worry well founded? She thought, "A mother's heart always knows!" She smiled, sad at her own rightness. She hoped she would be proved wrong.

It happens all the time. People under extreme duress indulge in food. Being a foodie for a person with normal health may result in obesity but a kidney patients' life gets compromised. There's a food chart, for daily consumption of products with phosphorus, potassium and sodium. It the balance is disturbed, the consequence is beyond imagination.

Lucy's phosphorus levels rose high, confirmed by repeated blood evaluations. Much to her caretaker's consternation, she refused to take warning signals seriously.

Due to high blood phosphorous she suffered from common cardiovascular complications. In peritoneal dialysis even if done daily, it removes phosphorous from the body poorly. She was forced to change her diet by reducing phosphorus intake, additional phosphorus binders were introduced to bind phosphorus in the gut so that the body does not absorb the phosphorus.

But these measures were insufficient or late in coming. The fangs of hypophosphatemia and secondary hyperparathyroidism in its severe forms caught her. Doctors smoothed ruffled feathers saying, "This is worldwide recognized as most likely among dialysis patients."

Lucy slowly went into other complications including a larger heart, with poor functions. They inserted a defibrillator to prevent irregular heart rhythm and low blood pressure, but the device infected her heart. Miraculously after removing the device she got relief from an antibiotic therapy.

Her parathyroid condition had deteriorated so with a clinical procedure, 'parathyroidectomy' most of the glands were removed.

Through many years of changing lanes from high medical challenges, stable life, to another health calamity, Lucy's attitude to life underwent a change. Through the heavy cloud draping her in a fortress, she saw some light penetrate to give her life another reason to smile.

Year 2004, gave Lucy Canton her life's most precious gift. A kidney was transplanted.

Now, as a mother she should focus on coming events. Things that need to recorded as most memorable event… the wedding that unites Lucy with Robert. "I shouldn't be vulnerable to sad thoughts,' she kept reminding herself.

She had watched Lucy while the wail was being placed firmly on her head and had felt her heart flowing with happiness. At the church with excitement raising the pace of heartbeat, she had stood mesmerized seeing Lucy looking enthralled with happiness. She experienced a unique moment of happiness. She wiped a tear and prayed for happy times for Lucy and Robert.

Time went by. Lucy came home less often. The mother reprimanded herself, "I must realize Lucy has new responsibilities! A husband to care." She thought of the dark days of the past sometimes with sadness and at other times sent a silent prayer upwards.

And then one day over lunch she reminded Lucy of her follow-up tests. Lucy smiled, "Oh yes, I must do it, will do it soon, Mom!" But from Lucy's tone, she was not convinced about the earnestness.

Next morning, the mother took her window seat and the beads between her fingers were moving, slowly now as her heart was submerged in a familiar fear.

A few months later, her fear became real.

Lucy had lost her kidney. Time for worry began. Now seriously.

> Families with kidney patients also go through the ordeals of the disease. Without actually experiencing dialysis or huge implications of a transplant parents are aware of the agony and feel sad for pain experienced by the person. It may be simply watching the child go through the pricks of the needle, seeing large volumes of blood circulating in the dialyser and wondering what does it feel to have the water, fluids, blood move around disturbing their child's peace. It's seeing the person's frown, expression of frustration and trying to fathom the extent of sorrow. Lucy's mother was extremely sensitive to even a feather touch on Lucy and dedicated caregiver.
>
> Kidney transplants give back opportunity to lead normal lives. But it is a package deal. With the new kidney, new responsibilities need to be shouldered. There's simply no way to take it lightly. Body shows symptoms early enough. One needs to catch signs and get back to the doctor and clinic immediately.
>
> Sadly for Lucy, it was too late. Very soon she began dialysis.

WHAT'S IN YOUR RED BAG? – RYAN GRIFFITH, UNITED KINGDOM

RG, that's what friends called him and he loved it that way. It was an evening birthday dinner and he had a Facebook friend asking many questions.

"By the way, which city are you from?"

"I'm from UK, not from the US!" he said teasingly.

"RG... tell me a little about your health".

"Oh, my health is a great secret. I need time to explain all the medical terms. You need to understand and appreciate my experience."

"I think RG you're being very possessive and want to hold tight."

He used the laugh smile and said later, tomorrow. He could see his wife was ready and they would be late.

"See you around later GS..."

Though she had a beautiful name, RG chose to call her by the initials.

As they rode to the party, RG's mind went back to the conversation.

"What should I talk about? Was GS going to understand all the different things I had in my bag?"

His wife saw him deep in thought and nudged her 70 year-old-husband. Without a preamble RG talked as if continuing an old conversation, "Remember how I was shocked by that collapse almost four decades back... I can't stop wondering why on earth it happened!

They held hands and walked into the party room. The evening was interesting and RG relaxed and mingled.

Late that night, after the party RG pulled out the *red bag* and reached out for the files. One was from 1972, with his merchant navy company's name and emblem. It had a sticker that read as "Accident".

He read the report out, "On duty a nasty accident with a 4 ton steel block, landing on his back. The initial x-rays showed Mild Lumbar Fracture. Patient was able to walk when discharged. Heavy doses pain killers have settled him."

"That's their summation. But then what happened next showed no evidence of connection to the accident."

"And... the pain killers stayed with me," he smiled sadly.

The second file was from 1986. It read Occupational Asthma.

RG read the report, softly now as it was well after midnight and he didn't want to disturb his wife. "It is an occupational lung disease, a kind of asthma. There's inflammation in the airway, reversible airways obstruction, and bronchospasm. It may be due to environment at workplace.

Rx – symptoms include coughing, wheezing, shortness of breath, some tightness in chest area. Some mild nasal involvement seems to be there."

He remembered how angry he was with this! Were they two connected? Accident and occupational asthma actually due to the accident! Nobody made this theory.

Then he picked up the 1993 file – "Hiatus Hernia" he read in a tired voice.

Another lousy one! More of a nuisance! Slowly, opening the file he read what he had scribbled on the inner flap, "An inner body part pushed itself and occupied some other area giving rise to an hiatus hernia."

Then he read the report, "Observed an opening in the diaphragm separating the esophagus from the chest. The esophagus passing through the hiatus has connected to the stomach. The stomach is pushing towards the chest."

Rx-Proton pump inhibitors (PPIs) prescribed to reduce the acid in the stomach.

They are commonly used to treat acid reflux, stomach ulcers and part of the gut called the duodenum. Most people who take a PPI do not develop any side effects.

"Another journey of sorts now began with more medications piling on my counter!" he said amused.

"Ah, there it is. The secret one I was thinking about while chatting with GS!"

Pulling it out of the bag his eye caught the big red??? on the cover.

His fore finger, ran over the figure and he drew a deep breath.

"What a great let down! Suddenly I discovered that my kidneys were losing their function and I was with chronic kidney disease. Apparently my doctors felt not too concerned so never spoke about it."

RG's eyes grew moist with tears. His mind went through the past events..."*They noticed and didn't tell me or they never really studied my report in detail to notice it? Was I too busy or too much in pain to not see where my health was going?"*

Wiping his eyes he reprimanded himself, "Why hurt when nothing is reversible in life!"

After five minutes of sitting quietly taking charge of his emotions, he picked up the last file.

In 2015 his health had gone down and he was rushed to the hospital in an emergency condition. Many tests were done over the next few days and finally *Multiple Myeloma* - cancer of the plasma cells and Chronic Lymphocytic Leukemia – blood and bone marrow cancer were both detected. Immediately they scheduled several cycles of chemotherapy.

Between the cycles RG developed a heart problem. So right in midst of the confused state of health he underwent a double heart stent operation.

Finally the chemotherapy came to an end.

Heaving a sigh of relief, RG's had smiled and suggested to his wife, "I had enough of drama and could do with a holiday!"

She loved the idea and had spread her arms out!

But the doctors somehow had extraordinary energy and they suggested a stem cell transplant as next treatment for remission!

Recalling what happened next, RG said, "How despairing it was! My nephrologist turned it down as with my kidney condition it was not appropriate!"

An accidental discovery of CKD and the rejection of a stem cell transplant was a sad culmination of how far CKD could impact.

Ryan Griffith

Red bag got its' contents purely by accident. One seems to have lead to another. All of them beyond any mathematical calculation! In the 1970's medical prescriptions were different. Long term use of medications are said to cause CKD. So the numerous files found their mysterious way into one bag.

MARIA'S BABY WAS SAVED! – MARIA ROMANO

Changes in life for 22-year-old Maria Romano seemed constant. But after a long time this one made her very happy. As she tried to overcome the emotional moment with tears flowing down her beautiful cheeks, her right hand gently pressed her abdomen looking for a lightening connect with the little one residing there. Her lips parted softly calling out, "Sweetheart".

Hendric Romano wove his arm through her arms to hold her close to him. He knew this was the ultimate joy of their life. He brushed her cheeks gently, wiping away traces of tears and they laughed in happiness.

Slowly they walked towards their car. "Where shall we celebrate?"

Maria eyes shone brightly as she said, "Brunch Place", lets enjoy our usual Sunday brunch in advance."

Hendric started his car and whistled softly through the ride. Suddenly his brow creased and his eyes grew grave. An hour later they would go to the Dialysis Center. That was Maria's thrice a week routine. Today it would be difficult! Maria will suddenly be facing the whole truth. So happiness was this ride, the brunch and….

Maria was chattering away, "So unexpected this is! I never dreamt of this!" She talked of the baby and how they need to do detailed planning. Her excitement was infectious and Hendric joined in the conversation trying to keep the upbeat mood.

But it was when Maria began dialysis that she faced reality.

"Am I allowed this? As a kidney patient getting pregnant could cause complications! Should I have talked to my nephrologist before?"

Slowly nervousness set in, after an hour or so sadness crept in and she was sobbing softly. The attending nurse noticed this and paged the psychologist.

The elderly matron-kind psychologist walked down the hallway and hailed to Maria. Maria's agitated face tried a smile and the matron took a chair for a chat. "Is everything alright Maria?" she asked gently.

With some effort and prompting Maria shared her latest news. Soon the nurse and technicians stopped by to congratulate her. Soon she regained her composure.

A few days later she met her nephrologist.

Opening her file, the doctor read, "22 years old, developed chronic kidney disease secondary to IgA nephropathy. She had irregular menstrual periods."

"So young lady, now your pregnancy report confirms it." He looked up smiling. Then reaching out to lightly pat her shoulder he said, "Lets handle it properly. It is important to watch your vitals and be careful on medications so you have an easy delivery."

Over the next few months she was given extra schedules of dialysis. The fluid balance was monitored; blood pressure was watched and treated; correction of anemia with intravenous iron and erythropoietin therapy. The pregnancy was full term and she delivered with C-section.

"I always told you pregnancy is safe, if well managed. It simply needs close monitoring! You're a good patient," the nephrologist's tribute brought smile to her tired lips. "Thank you, so much doctor. You protected my child!"

In Maria's case talking to her doctor made her pregnancy easy. Good and continuous health monitoring saved the baby. Pregnancy for patients of IgA nephropathy is considered as "high risk" as levels of blood pressure or anemic conditions could affect the baby's development. It needs working closely with the nephrologists and being compliant with medical advice and directions given.

I'LL STAY ON DIALYSIS – RUTH REAGAN

The doctor was studying the annual test results of a twenty year old, Ruth Reagan. He remembered her from the previous visit as a happy and fun loving person. She would be the last patient that evening.

With a soft knock, Ruth entered through the door. With a smile the doctor greeted her starting conversation, "How are you?" Ruth smiled and responded with honesty,

"Doctor, I am well, but tired after a long day at school".

The doctor smiled and continued, "I am sure. But, Ruth I have here results of the blood test. There is reason for you to slow down. The high blood pressure is a worry and it is noticed that your kidneys are functioning poorly. The kidney function could deteriorate with passage of time."

With a sinking heart she heard him talk about aggressive control of blood pressure to preserve her kidney function, significant change of life style, getting more active physically, dietary limitations and the medication regimen to control blood pressure. She decided to do it all.

Four years later, dialysis became necessary to sustain life. She understood merits of both peritoneal and hemodialysis treatment, which of these was an effective therapy for failed kidneys. She preferred to receive hemodialysis in-center three times a week and 3-4 hours each time. Ruth needed a creation of dialysis shunt in her arm for dialysis treatment.

Through this period Ruth stood determined chose receiving treatment as against not receiving treatment; accepted significant limitations in life style as against inviting death. She desired to live no matter what.

In her words, "I faced my share of dialysis and non-dialysis related complications. Sometimes it was revisions of dialysis shunts, suddenly shots of pain from a severe bone disease, abnormal heartbeats, even facial paralysis. But my twenty years into dialysis with reasonably stable condition is encouraging." As an after thought she added, "I will never consider trading my current condition with the other alternative. In fact I am now promoting this treatment for stable life for a kidney patient".

> Though transplant is an option offered to many people based on their chance of a good life post transplant and if chance of recurrence of the disease is not likely. People medically unfit for a transplant must choose to be positive even on dialysis.
>
> Ruth was very happy to remain on dialysis, due to several reasons. Many people make such a choice as they do not want anyone to sacrifice a kidney to save them or who are scared to face a failed transplant. Handling kidney disease and several aspects of the disease needs plenty of courage and an ability to withstand pressures and fight all odds. At every stage the disease keeps a person actively involved in healthcare. Neglecting any aspect at any stage is playing with fire. Early stages, with proper diet and medications kidney failure can be postponed for several decades. While on dialysis many danger zones emerge, as will be seen from many narratives in the book. Life on a transplant has management issues.
>
> After all, this disease is for a lifetime.

FEAR OF THE WHITE COAT –
SUBODH MUKHERJEE

Subodh Mukherjee studied the laboratory report as he walked out of the clinic. The high level of creatinine caught his eye.

2.0 mg/dl when normal range of creatinine was 0.6-1.2 mg/dl.

"Now what's going on?" he wondered a little worried about this rise. He met his doctor, Dr Lal who suggested that he meet a nephrologist. It was a disturbing thought.

In 1991, during a medical test, he had been alerted about his blood pressure being very high. It was in the range of 180/100. The same doctor had prescribed him blood pressure medication, which he had religiously taken for several years. Fear of any further health related news, had made him compliant with his medications. Without going back to the doctor he had managed to renew his prescriptions without much problem.

Married to Moushmi and with his kids very young, he believed he had managed his health well and with responsibility.

But now in 1999, as he turned forty years, things seemed to have changed. This blood test report was a shocker! The Indian doctor had also hinted that he lost 50% of its function.

That evening, over a cup of tea he shared his concerns with Moushmi, "There's some problem... remember the blood test I did? So... there's protein in the blood... creatinine is going up and Dr Lal said almost 50% of the kidney functions are gone!"

"What? Kidney failure?" she shouted as if she was hit by a rock.

"Not yet... but it will in some time?"

"What does Dr Lal want you to do?"

"Go to a nephrologist, a kidney specialist!"

Moushmi sat still. She knew it was a tough situation. Subodh had a phobia about doctors, hospitals. He would joke with her, "I suffer from 'white coat syndrome'!"

She was worried for her family.

In August 2003, Subodh's legs were swollen so when he went to the doctor, a blood test revealed that creatinine had risen to 8 mg/dl. For a better lifestyle he was put on to peritoneal dialysis. The surgery for placing the catheter in the peritoneum cavity faced a problem, so a second surgery was needed.

PD worked well for him. But he faced some very unusual experiences.

In Dec 2005, he went with his family to India to attend a family wedding. While fixing his seat belt the metal buckle was accidentally resting on top of the exit site. This pressure caused the cusp to leak.

Such an incident is avoidable, but when it happens it causes panic and one can just feel so unsure of life. Getting back to the doctor to change the catheter was critical. It was not that Subhod didn't learn from his mistake, but when he had another incident he was terrified.

In Nov 2008, while on the treadmill with a 1000CC of fluid dwelling, the bouncing of the fluid caused the exit site to leak. The leak continued for sometime leading to a severe peritonitis. This meant his catheter needed to be replaced. For some time he had to stay on hemodialysis. Both these episodes showed how much being on PD one can easily take things for granted and be complacent. Subodh felt these could have been avoided.

Mousmi had said, "Maybe you should have opted for the transplant when the call came 2005!"

Subhod could not remind her of his concern for the kids' education. They were still in school. So he sought a postponement. But he knew that it was the best decision for him.

Finally January 2009 brought about a change in life. He had his transplant.

His own assessment on his health:

- My first test in 1991, showed high blood pressure. Thereafter, I went to get refill from the pharmacy without checking my blood pressure.
- I should have done periodical blood tests and monitored my blood pressure.
- In 1999 when Dr Lal suggested I meet a nephrologist, I should have followed his advice. The nephrologist may have changed my medicines and even increased dosage to keep my BP under control.
- I was comfortable with the refills, which meant not meeting a doctor. Fear of meeting a doctor who will tell me about my serious health, made me lose my kidney. Limited vision of life and the belief that I could live life as per my terms was my greatest tragedy. With great humility I have understood that one must open doors to wisdom and never allow fear to manage our life.
- The belt's buckle damaging my dialysis catheter or exercising on a treadmill that affects the catheter's exit site due to the abdomen's muscle movement seem too small to think about. These so called small mistakes in reality costs so much pain and unwanted complications. In dialysis both big and small things need to understood and taken into consideration.

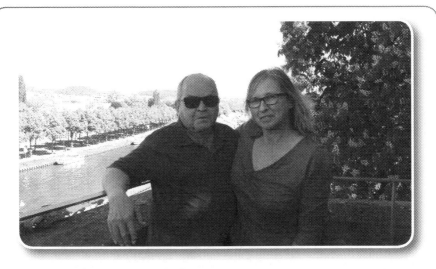

FORTY-SEVEN YEARS OF VALUABLE DIALYSIS EXPERIENCE – THOMAS LEHN, GERMANY

Today, I Thomas Lehn can say I'm the longest survivor on hemodialysis in the whole world. There is no pride in living so long with this treatment but to stand testimony to changes in medical advancement makes me wonder at Lord choosing for me this life.

I recall clearly, I had just turned 14 years and I faced shocking experiences about my health and life. I want to share with you an abstract of the worst time of my life as episodes that I can clearly remember, even today:

On 20 of August 1970 I was deadly sick, temporarily disoriented, blind, extraordinarily high blood pressure, my small body filled with over 10 liters of water. I lay in the intensive care unit of the Surgical Clinic in Heidelberg. Late Dr. Hans Wolf Schueler, a physician and urologist held my hand. He checked my left hand first, then my right arm searching for blood vessels. For several minutes with great concentration he closed his eyes, then declared, that I would not die, of the uremic toxins and the fluids in my body. He would put me into emergency surgery as soon as possible to fix a Scribner-Shunt.

This became the first step for my first dialysis.

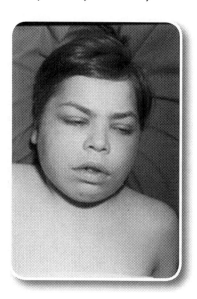

My condition being so bad, I couldn't see him, but I could hear him say. "Head up my boy, we will manage this. We will be set you up with this. Please be brave, you will live!"

Dead or alive

It was the early rays of the sun that awoke me up. I stretched myself and felt constricted. Looking around I saw some tubes and the walls white walls. I recollected about my being in a hospital after being diagnosed with terminal kidney insufficiency. It had seemed as if I was awarded a death sentence. During the 1970's dialysis was not so advanced and few people were lucky to get treated. *(Today, in developing countries and economically poor countries patients still face such conditions and feel insecure)*

Many things were wrong. I was young, far away from family and I suffered multi morbid conditions. I felt more dead than alive! For many days I was in the small room of the Surgical University Clinic at Heidelberg and that too at an infernal dialysis machine. I can't remember how many days and nights I was on dialysis. It was possible that only because of Valium I could survive 12 hours of dialysis. I never noticed, when another kid next to me had dialysis and who fought for life or succumbed to death. That was the bitter choice: death or life!

I recall there were two dialysis units and even in those days we had 10 children below 14 years. So with a round the clock shift the kids got turns to get dialysis. Sadly a new kid was admitted to the dialysis program only when a space became available or when a patient died. Sometimes I sit and wonder how the doctors and nurses worked so hard with mental stress. It was true about the first few hours of admission.

After three sessions of dialysis I felt better. By now about 8 liters of fluid and the high concentration of the uremic substances were removed from my body. Surprisingly all this by a rustic, Travenol dialysis machine, which stands no comparison to today's advanced and more effective dialysers and machine.

And then, yes, my eyes could see my mother again, who visited me every day.

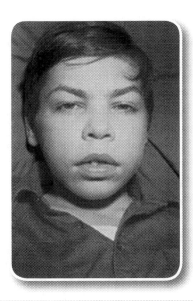

After 12 hours of dialysis, I wasn't able to walk upright in the first hours. The next day I would rest. I was mostly very ill, so I was brought to Children's Hospital by ambulance or I woke up in an emergency room and would go later back to the children's hospital.

Children dialysis – a big experience

Today everyone talks of complications. Back then nobody knew, what kind long-term complications could be expected in children. They knew that in relation to adult patients, children have unstable blood vessels. Would the young organism tolerate the strenuous hemodialysis duration? How would young patients grow up? Does dialysis affect the metabolism and hormone levels in children? Would the dialysis filter away hormones, especially growth hormones? Will children come into puberty? Will they be able to lead an independent life in future? Will they be able to have a normal education and pursue a career along with getting dialysis treatment? Is the Scribner shunt a permanent connection for hemodialysis? What problems could occur on the long way? It is possible to live a normal live with transplantation?

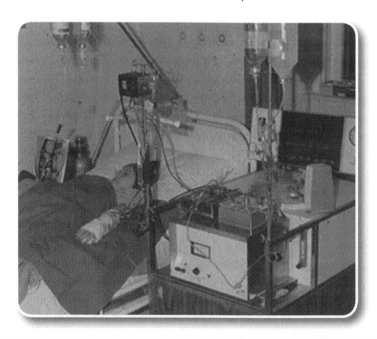

There were thousands of questions, but nobody knew an answer at that time. It was such a visual and learning experience.

Better technology, shorter dialysis time!

Over time, the dialysis machines grew better and were a lifesaver!

New dialyzers called Capillar artificial kidneys were developed. They cleaned the blood better and faster. Another good development came with 2008S from Fresenius, which had a ultrafiltration. This new machine with ultrafiltration volume shouldered many health issues to bring patients' comfort and ease. It could calibrate weight gained and lost. The standard machine included a heparin pump that could help you control the fragmin or heparin. By bicarbonate dialysis treatment was better and gentle as the acetate dialysis, known previously. Gambro AK5 as it was called was the most modern dialysis machine with good electronic features. This gave freedom for dialysis staff to care for others who needed care. Alarms triggered if there is something wrong with the machine's working condition or patient is threatened of any danger. The Dialysis schedule hours got reduced to 2x10 hours, then to 3x8 hours per week.

From Tommy to Thomas

During the years I used my dialysis time trying to understand the medical and technical advancement in dialysis and gather medical knowledge. My thirst for knowledge about my illness made me question doctors and nurses, who were really very helpful. I depended on them for information, as the Internet was non-existent.

I got my education with teachers help as a guest-student in the school. I completed my education ultimately with success, with my high school leaving certificate. My youth was not much different, from my healthy young friends.

In1975 I meet my Beate. We were in love. In 1978 I got trained as a computer programmer. October 1980 I took my job. I am still in employment there for 37 years employed as a systems engineer.

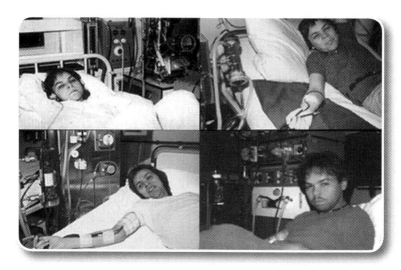

Home hemodialysis

In 1983 I began the home hemodialysis. In1984 we got married.

I decided against the transplantation, because I discovered home hemodialysis as most perfect treatment and most suitable renal replacement therapy for me.

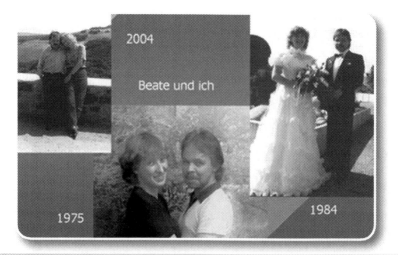

Travel and dialysis worldwide

Beate and I love to travel, and we've stayed at many places all over the world with dialysis treatment. Today it is possible to go on dialysis holidays all over the world. We were in Egypt, Turkey, South Africa, USA, Domrep, Greece, Mexico, Jamaica, Canarya Islands, Croatia, etc.

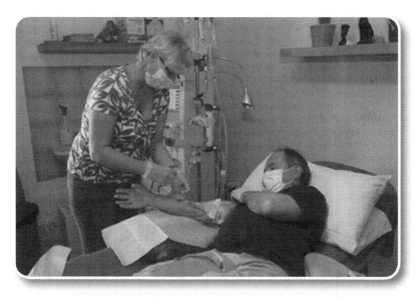

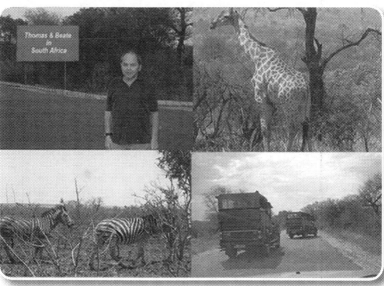

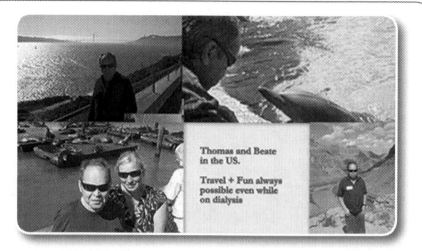

Thomas and Beate
in the US.

Travel + Fun always
possible even while
on dialysis

Kidney transplant, not my cuppa

In early years I evaluated transplant options. Some health issues gave me reason to avoid it. By choosing home dialysis I grew more comfortable. Over the years my views on kidney transplant changed.

My opinion is: when my body will accept a foreign organ only with the use of medications, called immunosuppressants and which can decrease the immune defense and will continue to fight all my life not letting the organ be considered as part of my body makes me feel sad. In addition, the transplanted organ is always exposed to renal failure. The immunosuppressive agents in the body set free autonomous processes that neither medicine nor I have any control, makes me uncomfortable.

I am not against transplantation, but will accept it if all possible components of a transplant are clarified. And, yes, I'm not registered for a kidney transplant.

How do I manage?

I know that my health has been managed as I give attention to certain rules. I am certain that when I refuse foods with high phosphate and potassium, I'm fine. When I don't drink so much, take my prescribed medication (Vitamin d, phosphate binder and so on) I'll be fine. If I follow my long dialysis routine of 6 hours and more, stick to a frequency of three to four times in the week, I'll be fine. For me it is very important to have good medical consultants. I also want to be properly informed. The social environment is important. Family and friends need to accept that dialysis comes with a baggage of additional diseases. With all these components and compromises with co-operative my wife I try to lead an almost normal life – and hoping it will last for a long, long time.

My basket of complications:

In 47 odd years I have seen many problems touch, pierce and go. It matters to me, but I know baskets have things some of which are not our choice. My bones are damaged by the long-term dialysis, which is based on the chemical process of calcium-phosphate metabolism in the kidney. I have often bone pain and joint pain. My parathyroid glands were removed 28 years ago. Five years back I had carpal tunnel syndrome surgery on both hands. Sometimes neuropathy in the legs, amyloidosis in the right foot are fairly predictable, but not to be underestimated. I am satisfied with my health and I hope that I can continue to hold on to my conditions.

My life motto: *The life is strong but beautiful!* Live your dreams as long as you can.

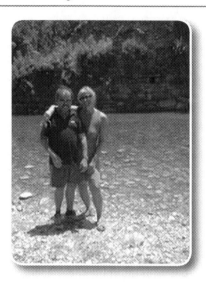

Thomas Lehn
Bergstrasse 30
55218 Ingelheim
Germany
web: http://www.thomas-lehn.de or http://www.dialyseshunt.com
mail: Thomas.Lehn@online.de

COMPLICATIONS WITH LUPUS
– SALINA GABRIEL

Salina cried out in anguish, "Mom, why is this pain in my joints not subsiding? It tires me so much. And... this skin rash all over the body also bothers me. What's gone wrong with me?"

Her mother examined the rash and was worried about the rapid spread. She knew of some good local remedies that were available, so she purchased some for Salina's use.

But the rash was so adamant that it continued to show on Salina's skin leaving her unhappy.

In 1983, Salina Gabriel was a16 year-old carefree teenager who pursed her education, enjoyed life with her family and did all those fun-things that one does in their youth. But when she suffered from these joint pains, which were in her hands, her upper and lower extremities she was depressed! It ached all the time! She tired easily. She struggled to perform normal routine activities, when her friends burst with energies and liveliness.

"Mom, what's happening? I feel so very lousy! I have lost 98lbs in just a few months. How can there be so much happening!" she said as she just broke down under the enormous weight of this unknown disease.

Her mother had noticed her weight reduction and Salina's skeletal look bothered her too!

Gradually other things piled up. Salina was bothered about her lack of appetite, her low energy levels even to feed myself! And then, the blood test showed her nutrition levels dropped lower than required for a healthy body. Local remedies failed to revive her health, and suddenly it dawned on mother-daughter that her deteriorated would need medical consultancy from a doctor.

The doctor immediately hospitalized. Salina went into comatose, remaining in that state for three days. In the intensive care unit, she was hooked onto a heart monitoring equipment. Her large family and friends were worried, prayed fervently showing their support and visiting her in the hospital. Her boy friend suffered from uncontrollable pangs of sorrow seeing Salina in such a critical condition.

When Salina came out of coma, the attendant doctor disclosed result of investigations. She had Lupus an autoimmune disease that could become very dangerous. The doctor explained the disease and the line of treatment, involving some powerful medications to control the disease. Though these drugs had serious side effects they were essential for treating the disease and preventing its progression.

Two months stay in the hospital, with best of treatment from the doctors brought Salina back to her feet. But for the next three years Salina was occupied with fighting the disease. She was tormented with a low blood count, aching joints, facial rash, high blood pressure, fevers, muscular pain, hair loss, mouth ulcers, and fatigue.

For a teenager it was tough to handle all these miseries and in her depressed state Salina frequently fought temptation of committing suicide. To add to the complications she developed salmonella infection after consuming some snake pills from a local pharmacy.

Soon her kidneys showed signs of failing. Treatments were started, with chemotherapy being the first line of treatment. But Salina was unable to tolerate beyond three sessions of chemotherapy. In some time, when her levels of creatinine rose high and kidneys failed she began dialysis.

After a year and eight months, Salina received her twin sister's kidney so that she did not become dialysis dependent and enjoyed a reasonably good life. But through this new phase of life, Salina was concerned about her sister's well being.

The kidney transplant was successful. Salina took her medications religiously, though her face looked like chipmunk. She wanted to care for her prized kidney possession. She got married and within four years from the kidney transplant she had a baby girl. By now Salina had got used to a reasonably comfortable life and the lupus was in remission. Her sister was also in good health.

But in Salina's life things were never peaceful. Three years later she was divorced and a month later she was diagnosed with cancer of vulvar. After nearly 25 biopsies, of which five revealed she had cancer, and the need for undergoing three extensive surgeries were established and the oncologists were advising to remove the cancerous growth.

Twelve years later Salina is grateful for being free of cancer.

After completing seventeen years with the transplanted kidney transplantation, she chose to stop her immunosuppressant medication. Her daughter, now a teenager and is her source of joy. Salina continuous fighting stress and depression, that surfaces now and then.

> Lupus is such a rare autoimmune disease that people are overwhelmed with its' unexpected ways of impacting health. The fact that it can flare up anytime and sometimes lead to multiple organ failure keeps people on tenterhook. Living with Lupus is tough but medical advancements has made survival a reality if there's an opportunity to get treated and manage many conditions arising due to the disease.

DIABETES PLAYED TRUANT – JOSÉ THOMAS

Jose Thomas sat in the restaurant. He had ordered a small meal. Many things were not permitted now, with his restricted diet. Twelve years ago, at this same place he had met her. He sat back with his memories.

The music floated around the fully occupied restaurant. People ordered their meal and chatted mostly. At the far end, she was dipping into her favorite garlic chicken pasta, sipping wine and enjoying the soulful music. Jose, the lead singer was a jubilant young man and his band played at several restaurants on special invitation. He made it a point to go round and chat with people after the session. This gave the evening certain warmth, and was much appreciated by the regulars at the joint.

The applause was loud as he completed the last song for the evening.

"Thank you friends, for being such a great audience," Jose said, waving both arms alternatively.

Though he was overweight, he was a happy man, content with life and his music.

Jose recalled that evening. "I remember that kind lady was sitting at this very table. She had praised me for my wonderful spirit." Then shrugging his shoulders, he sat sipped water he was wondering what his future be. "My wonderful life was simply cut short, it just came tumbling down," he murmured as if in a trance.

He chuckled at the unanticipated changes that had happened to his life.

It had begun with a few conditions that didn't seem serious at all. He had faced fatigue, which even after a good night's sleep didn't seem to vanish. Friends had asked him to lose weight and do strenuous exercise. But being so overweight meant even starting any exercise was a humungous task!

When he had become irritable with his general health he had seen a doctor. After a few preliminary check-ups, he was directed to a laboratory for a few blood tests. He was diagnosed with type-2 diabetes that grew into the much dreaded kidney failure.

This setback had come with several responsibilities! Now he needed to be regular on dialysis, had dietary restrictions and had to learn how to maintain a reasonable life style.

But all this went on smoothly for a brief spell. Jose's health continued to deteriorate. With peripheral neuropathy and vascular disease setting in, it became difficult for him to perform normal activities. So on many aspects his output was significantly limited. The greatest misfortune was the stroke, which affected his speech threatening his professional life. Jose felt very demoralized and depressed.

Smaller irritants with his dialysis stunt had meant multiple revisions to make it functional. The effects of peripheral vascular disease took its toll, as he had to undergo amputations of part of index of right hands and toes of left foot because of poor circulation and on set of gangrene.

These complications accompanied pain, infections of lower extremities, frequent hospitalizations, visits to the orthopedics and other specialists. Life changed dramatically; he could not drive to dialysis and he lost control over his health.

Jose knew in his heart that without support of his sister he could never survive. She was such a great motivator that she could revive his zest to live a reasonable life.

Reflections: The 'early detection' is much talked about and emphasized today. It is well known obesity could bring about many health complications. Unless a person takes early action this is where life could go. Managing diabetes with medications, diet and exercise can save a person if diabetes is detected early.

Monitoring all aspects of health thereafter is the only way to sail through disease. Strictly following physician's advice and keeping faith on treatments is most important. Diabetes has no known cure. It can only be treated.

Jose Thomas

DETERMINATION MAKES HER WIN!
– MARY SLONE

Mary Slone was discussing with friends on career options one evening. When they turned to her to understand which career was of her interest, she surprised them. "I want to be a pharmacist. It's a very good way to understand quality of medicines, somewhere you get to ensure that they are properly made available, lawfully." All her friends were impressed with her ambitious plans. The twenty-year-old was very aspiring and a very loving person, so universally loved.

One evening when getting ready for a family dinner, she noticed a butterfly rash on her cheeks. It kept bothering her that it was on the face and marring her looks.

Conscious of her appearance she consulted a dermatologist who diagnosed it as lupus, an autoimmune disease. She was prescribed medications including *plaquanil* and *imuran* to control her disease. But the disease flared us gradually progressively affecting her blood, joints, and led to a kidney failure.

She had just graduated from college and was admitted by the USC Pharmacy School. She made a very considered choice of peritoneal dialysis that would give her time to study and take control of her health. While others in her institute could focus on their studies and enjoy a carefree life, Mary's had no time for any social life.

To be par with her classmates, she required working very hard. Significant time was spent on peritoneal dialysis and she was regular with clinic visits, so she could monitor her medical condition and have follow-up meetings with her kidney specialist. None of this came in the way of her achieving her goal.

"Congratulations, Pharmacist Mary! You conquered Lupus!" her physician welcomed her into the clinic with a huge smile. On his table was a cake. "We need to celebrate. "You're one of my best patients. Many people leave school as if CKD means end of life. But Mary you never succumbed to any external pressures," he concluded. It was a happy hour with the doctor who encouraged her always, with kind words. It was an emotional moment for Mary. But back home too there was a huge celebration.

Her heart swelled with happiness. Mary had become a pharmacist!

Through her life she faced unexpected trials, leaving her sometimes depressed. But it was with great grit she fought those moments and never let hope for survival leaves her side. Mary's deep faith, family support and encouragement she received from her kidney specialist and nurses enabled her to meet new challenges courageously. In her success all of them participated with joy!

Further treatments of immunosuppressant therapy and other relevant medications were given as required. Despite multiple blood pressure medications, her blood pressure was uncontrollable. She was hospitalized due to a massive stroke, requiring assisted ventilation and stroke management in the ICU.

The worst after effect of the stroke was, she could no longer continue with her peritoneal dialysis. So after five years Mary moved into hemodialysis so that there was need to cope with catabolic state, and management of severe electrolyte and fluid balance.

While in ICU, Mary was treated by a group of physicians including a neurologist. Revival from coma seemed a remote possibility, but the family and her kidney specialist didn't leave any stone unturned. Unexpectedly she made recovery. After weeks of hospitalization in the acute hospital and two months in rehabilitation center, her condition returned to normalcy.

On hemodialysis for about two years Mary is stable and has no clinically detectable residual neurologic deficit. Soon she is expected to receive her license to practice. She is aware that dialysis is her lifeline and prefers peritoneal over hemodialysis, though she would love to rather live without it. She is eagerly awaiting her chance for kidney transplantation.

Sheer determination helped Mary to manage Lupus and complete her dream education. In chronic kidney disease it has commonly been found as if a trait in youth and young adults that they quit education and lucrative jobs, many times encouraged by family elders. Such actions spur out of deep fear of loss of life as managing the disease is very difficult. Value of finishing one's education and keep a job that generates income has to be subtly promoted to patients and their family members. Everything rests on the patient's shoulders. Disease management is better when the person is emotionally positive and strives to overcome the disease and all limitations supposedly placed by it.

One needs emotional boost, encouragement and sufficient resources to take care of unexpected treatment costs. Mary was passionate about her career so she secured herself sufficiently to face the disease and medical costs. People around her were impressed and they would be willing donors who would support her survival plans.

YOU CAN SET YOUR OWN BOUNDARIES
– JIMMY MCGRAW

Jimmy McGraw was a man with a happy disposition. Life had to be lived fully without any curb on his hikes. The joy of outdoor always excited him. Working as a civil engineer in a top-notch building construction company, also added scope for his travel. He did amazing work as a engineer and was quite a favorite among family and friends.

And when he retired from work in 1973, the recreation time got extended beyond everybody's imagination! Friends were amazed with his energy and as much as they tried, they failed to match to his zest. He enjoyed a very fruitful life with a large family five sons, five daughters, many grand children and great grand children. He travelled widely to 47 states within the US, Mexico, and Canada, making each trip exciting, and a memorable experience as he drove in RV's.

It was sometime in the end of 2002, that he developed subtle symptoms suggestive of coronary artery disease. Coronary angiogram confirmed serious coronary disease and he underwent quadruple bypass. Unfortunately, this got complicated into a congestive heart failure and his kidneys also quit working. He was referred to a kidney specialist for further evaluation.

"Jimmy, much as I hate to say, though your physical condition has improved and you are feeing fit and strong, your kidneys are damaged. You will need to start dialysis very soon."

Jimmy declined the kidney specialist's recommendation to start dialysis. Adopting persuasive and rational methods the specialist convinced the ninety-year old gentleman to try out dialysis before making any long-term decision.

This strategy proved successful. After his first dialysis Jimmy felt more energetic and gradually he maintained the schedule given by the doctor. As soon as health improved Jimmy used his boyish charm to convince the doctor to permit him a weekend break when he would travel on his RV.

On the RV he has his regular escapades traveling around the country. He is active, walks short distances and gets political news updates on television. At ninety-six years he has been on dialysis for more than 5 years.

Though Jimmy never liked dialysis, which he believed compromised his freedom he never got depressed and he is compliant with medications and diet to the satisfaction.

> Healthy mind maketh healthy body. With kidney disease not much on health improvement can be achieved. But being happy through dialysis takes away burden of the disease and reduces sorrow. Jimmy's escapades made living with dialysis far easier.

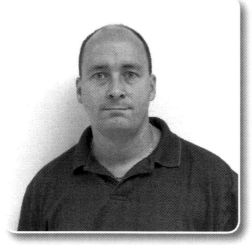

Eric Lee (Altruistic Donor)

RARE, HEAVENLY ENCOUNTER

Under a thick layer of bed covers, Eric rolled restlessly. His face was distorted with stress, even as beads of sweat broke on his forehead, sending strong early signals. In a few minutes he kicked his strong legs struggling to break loose. As the agitation increased, he sat up, shaking compulsively, bed sheets thrown away. Mona stirred in bed, eyes still heavy with sleep she murmured, "What's up hon...ey?"

Eric's heavy breathing, escaping from his lips noisily, was enough for Mona to stir out of bed, sleep lingering on her heavy eye-lids. Eric's body was shaking violently.

Under the calming effect of her soft touch, Eric began gasping, slowly releasing his anguish. Mona poured out water and extended the glass to her husband. A few sips of water, seemed to help him calm a bit, but he spoke as if under the strain of a traumatic experience.

"It was a dream...so powerful, so real unlike any I have seen before."

"Tell me Eric," she coaxed him suppressing her own fears.

When Eric sat stunned looking straight ahead, she continued her attempt to break through his silence saying softly, yet firmly,

"Eric...all your life you dreamt such explosive dreams, sometimes of the past and others of a future...so what's new?"

"She is dying, you know and I need to help her soon, "Eric said nervously and he choked over his words.

"Eric, tell me exactly what happened!" Mona said in a firm tone, eyes filled with concern, while hand was gently stroking him. She knew Eric too well to take this dream lightly.

"I saw a woman... somehow I seemed to know her... as if we were friends. At first she looked fine... she appeared to be African American...that's what it seemed in there...in my dream," he looked at his wife to see if she believed him. She always did, but this one was somehow different.

"Her husband was a Caucasian, with a distinctly "funny" personality. She was very pleasant...but very quiet," Eric said reflectively.

"But something happened... suddenly I could sense that the atmosphere had changed, but didn't notice what made it so. Now, it was not any more friendly... it was sad and depressing all around. There was a visible change. I looked at my friend, saw her getting hooked up to a machine, with a connection on her arm, tubes leading from the machine stuck here" he pointed to his right arm below the elbow, looking at the place strangely as if needles were stuck there!

"When I looked up, I observed the change on her face. She looked very unhappy now and eventually I was no longer able to speak with her."

He paused. Then as if remembering the event and linking it to her sadness he said, "I saw her going for treatments several times. Plenty of treatment, I couldn't understand what was wrong with her.

"And then... I turned my head and saw myself lying in a pale blue hospital gown on a sterile, metallic operating table. The doctors were performing a surgery of some kind. I was lying still and there were doctors and nurses around. Then I saw vividly an incision on my lower left side, a long cut just below my waistline.

"And within minutes I saw my friend, receiving what they took from me," Eric looked peculiarly at his wife; puzzled or scared one couldn't understand from Eric's expression.

"What could it be...?" he asked into space hoping someone would give him a clue.

Mona had been watching him closely all through this time. She quickly prompted, "You need to write it down now. In the morning you can speak to a doctor, find out what that procedure was which you saw in your dream."

After some silence he talked, "I have recorded all my past dreams, when it is still fresh so...they are accurate. But this one....I hope...if it was possible to transfer what I have seen into visual transcripts that could be reproduced for display on a screen...it will be seen in true dimension, it was so real...just very scary!" He shook his shoulders as if to shoo the dream away.

"Tell me more, Eric," she goaded adding pressure by gripping his hand tighter.

"I never dwell on them too much, but always believed that many of my dreams had some link with my life, in some way."

"I know..." she said vaguely as her mind back to many such past dreams.

Now, fully aroused, Eric did just that. The next few days Eric spent in gathering information. He found out it was a laparoscopic surgery for a kidney transplant, which was least invasive that yielded a quick recovery. Less painful too!

He read about kidney disease, how patients suffer due to insufficient kidney function, restrictive diet, the morbidity of the disease and sufferance of patients.

Eric went into a frenzy digging deeper. He needed more relevant information. What did kidney patients need most? In the process he found out financial compensations were prohibited by Federal Law; contributions came by people giving time to conduct events which Eric had heard of before. The most significant was to give a part of oneself, unselfishly to bring about a dramatic change in a kidney patient's life; the trials experienced during dialysis, the long wait for allotment of a kidney; and ultimately the truth stood naked before him.

He should donate his kidney to someone, facing danger of extinction.

Eric discussed the organ donation with Mona and his two teenage daughters, in what was a heart rendering, overwhelming conversation. His earnestness while explaining the unique opportunity to help someone, sharing risk factors of the surgery and recovery and his concluding it as his heart's call, won him unilateral support for such an altruistic cause. It was his parent's worry that left Eric uncomfortable. Though he understood their concerns, he knew there was no way he would change his mind.

During the process of discussion his determination reached its peak.

Active search for a "worthy" patient began, with watching videos of people looking for a kidney donor. Eric was amazed at the simple process. Eric never knew anyone personally with a kidney disease, so now reading about left him horrified that large numbers lived in desperation. Mona and Eric found it extremely difficult to nail down a patient. Instead of finding the woman of his "dreams," he left it to God to find the right candidate.

One morning he walked into Yale New Haven Hospital met the transplant unit, offering to be a living donor. He expressed urgency to get the surgery done. Eric did not want any untoward incident to spoil this mission. With great speed a coordinator was allotted to Eric and process began.

The first piece of information that his blood group "O" meant his kidney could go to patients in any blood group, but if a person was with "O" he would be in desperate need as "O" blood group can only receive from another person with "O". Family understood its full implications that a person with "O" must be waiting long for a kidney.

In the months ahead, Eric played enthusiastically the game of donor evaluation more tests, scans, interviews (psychiatric & psychological), and physical examinations.

All this time, some 90 miles away from Connecticut, in Chestshire, Lisa was on a tight schedule with thrice a week dialysis. With great effort, every alternate week-day she dragged herself to the clinic. Being on dialysis for seven long years was having its toll. Her energy levels were gradually seeing a drop. But being very sensible she knew it was only way to survive.

One evening she returned home after a session and collapsed on the couch. Her husband Al was shocked to see her in such a state. He did everything to make her comfortable. But seeing her on slumped on the couch, had him worried; extremely worried.

That night as she lay in bed, every ounce of energy spent, she sent out a plea, "Lord, please find me a donor. This is how much I can manage to do."

Next morning, Lisa was clearing the breakfast table, while in a firm clasp she had a second cup of black coffee. Her mind was clouded with many thoughts, when the loud ring from the telephone, broke through her reverie.

The caller said, "Hey there, I am Susan Richard calling from the Yale New Haven Hospital. I need to speak to Lisa, please."

"Yes, this is Lisa."

"Hey Lisa, how are you doing? We have some good news for you. We have found a matching donor for you. Congratulations. Can you come over tomorrow at 11am to meet with the transplant team?"

With as much energy she could gather, Lisa said, "Yes, I will." Somewhere inside, she felt her heart was ready to burst, while the insides shrank nervously.

She fiddled with the phone and called Al.

"I got it Al. It's come. Hospital called. Tomorrow 11 am we need to meet."

In a few days, in early August Eric got a message, "We have found a recipient with a perfect match. The surgery date is fixed for 10th August."

Eric learnt it was a lady from Connecticut who was on dialysis for seven years.

It was a Tuesday morning, in spite of a bright sun smiling down, Eric was shivering with nervousness, but he was also excited.

As he finished the paperwork at the registration office, turning Eric saw a man wheeling a lady in a wheel chair. Struck by similarity, Eric said softly, "That's her." Mona turned, a bit too late, all she saw was a receding wheelchair going in the opposite direction.

In the recovery room Eric was informed that the surgery was successful.

Finally when he broke through the effects of anesthesia, Eric found himself in a room with happy smiling faces bending over him. Seeing his parents he knew that in spite of their initial hesitation, their faith in him remained intact.

In a few days, Eric returned to normal life. There was an extraordinary feeling of peace for having done given a body part, to change someone's way of life. He experienced some unusual moments of high, when he almost felt he was a soldier returning home from war.

Early December a letter came into his mailbox. Eric was completely taken aback. It was from Lisa. What she wrote was so soothing and unexpectedly tears of joy and excitement began to flow. She wanted to meet him!

Under the rules for kidney donation, he had agreed about not seeking his kidney recipient. But this was a happy surprise.

Closer to Christmas, Eric was invited by Lisa to her Christmas party. She called it a 'surprise' as she would not reveal to her the identity of the special festival guest.

The evening of the party, Eric found himself standing outside the main door, a bundle of nerves, excited. It took a moment and a deep breath, for him to knock on the heavy wood door.

As the door opened, Eric saw standing on the threshold the woman of his dream. Yes, it was her, the woman who had entered his dream, the very same person. The pieces of the puzzle fitted perfectly. It had been her all through, at the hospital on the wheelchair and in the adjacent operation theatre waiting for his kidney.

His eyes brimmed with tears, as this was something beyond his capacity to marvel, to understand and digest! The union was a very emotional experience for both of them, as they embraced a new relationship, called love. And, Lisa became part of Eric's extended family.

But now, Eric saw his role emerging as an advocate for organ donation. In the past few months, many aspects of the disease came to his consciousness that he could drive away from his mind. He was on warpath to spread word of the value of kidney donation.

As Eric came closer to Lisa, he learnt that Al had offered to donate his kidney, but due to a blood mismatch, the offer was turned down. Eric impressed upon Al to choose to donate to another patient in need.

Sometimes, when Eric recalls his dream his chest swells with pride. That, things fell into place, that he could manage to reenact the story as it unveiled itself in dream.

All he did was made a choice. It changed someone's life forever.

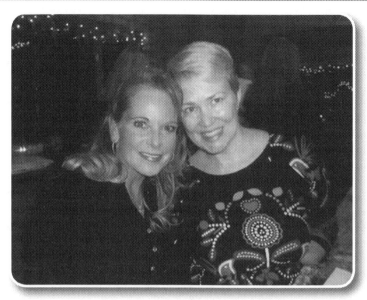

Left: Amy Otto (Altruistic Donor)
Right: Rebecca Springer (Transplantee)

STRIKING THE RIGHT CHORD

Amy Otto was busy scheduling official meetings for April.

Suddenly she stopped. "Oh! Becky's birthday is in April... How can I forget it," she bit her lower lip, reprimanding herself. She scribbled on her planner, "Becky's Birthday...gift to be ordered" and sat thinking of the fairly new friend, one who inspired her in more ways than one.

As she was drove home from work, she passed her favorite spa. In a flash, a fleeting thought turned into an interesting idea. Taking the service road, she maneuvered into an empty parking slot. Once inside the aromatic spa, she checked the packages they offered. Amy chose one she had used before and walked to the front desk ready to place the order. The manager at the desk smiled at Amy warmly, "Hey...How are you today?"

Amy smiled as she responded, "Hey...nice to see you. Wondering if you could spare a few moments? I want to buy a gift for a very dear friend, Becky Springer. I will fill the form, but need to speak to you and discuss some important aspects."

Taking her aside, Amy explained Becky's situation. From the change in expression in the

Manager's face, concern was evident as she quickly assured Amy. "Our customers find our personalized treatment awesome as we make it an ultimate joy for them. Your friend will be made completely at ease. She will enjoy it. I am very sure about that," she said bouncing her freshly trimmed bob, with added confidence.

Amy walked out overjoyed. What a perfect gift!

'Good...Becky needs to be pampered! She will simply love being in such a soothing, aromatic atmosphere. The fragrances...hmm,' she thought completely convinced no other gift would be better.

Amy was excited. "That's how I felt, wonderfully spoilt and pampered when Chuck surprised me with a spa gift last year." She grinned remembering her own exhilarating experience, the glow on her face when she walked into the restaurant for a romantic dinner later that evening. "Life is just a few moments of joy," she mused.

As she drove home, she recalled their first meeting, how the friendship had developed.

A book club of Mom's in an Atlanta suburb drew a group of women together monthly to discuss a book, enjoy wine and some good conversation floated around. Amy had been a part of the book club for about a year when they welcomed a new member, Becky.

Becky was gushing with life, smart and funny! She participated actively in the discussions, and her exuberance was infectious. It was easy for Amy to break ice with her. Soon they became good friends, sharing many common things. Their friendship was simply pure, unassuming, no strings attached. Amy admired Becky's capabilities and was astounded by her joy of life. Her interest in Becky was so heightened that she had taken every opportunity to know her closely.

She looked at the car mirror and smiled. Now their early days of friendship seemed so long ago. That evening as Amy was setting the dinner table, Chuck noticed Amy looking unexceptionally happy and raised his brows expectantly. Bubbling with eagerness she spoke of what she had done.

"Ah so you're planning Becky Springer's 'surprise' birthday gift," Andi chipped in from behind, winking at her brother while teasing her Mom. Between gurgles of laughter they recalled an earlier 'surprise gift' that had gone totally wrong. The dinner became hilarious with so many anecdotes of surprise parties and gifts.

But after dinner on a serious note, Amy narrated some major life changing events in Becky's life. On full stomach full, the family gave half an ear till the story reached its finale!

"It happened just after 2008's Valentine's Day. Becky felt a chill. She wore a cardigan when city temperatures were normal. That evening while trying to dial the phone, she realized her fingers had grown stiff; it simply would not flex. Alarmed, Paul had rushed her to the ER. She was admitted into the hospital for check-up.

The next morning when Becky came into consciousness a shattered Paul was trying to explain why...Till that time Becky was unaware that her hands and feet were no longer there! They were amputated in an emergency as the best resort under the circumstance. Can you predict her reaction?"

Amy stole a glance around. Now she saw them moving uneasily in their seats, as if they were roused. It's not that Amy anticipated any reaction other than surprise. Her eyes sparkled with pride as she continued pouring out the heart wrenching story, voice modulated to inspire her family,

"Unexpectedly Becky acted differently! She received the news calmly, unquestioningly. No wailing, no anger...none of the usual explosive behavior. Isn't that amazing! An anxious doctor explained to her the diagnosis. That Becky was a victim of Haemophilus Influenzae Type B, known as Hib.

"The terrible infection first attacked her organs. Kidneys were first to shut down. It led to

Septicemia, a serious, life-threatening condition caused by bacteria in her blood. A stroke was paralyzing her. To prevent further onslaughts by the infection, the hands and feet were sacrificed.

After six weeks at Rehabilitation Institute of Chicago, she regained her strength."It began with her on twenty-four hour dialysis, now reduced to thrice a week."

She sipped some water to calm her nerves and she concluded, "Back in Atlanta she continues with dialysis."

The family was stumped into silence. Becky's story was so startling, so unreal. Impossible to listen, understand and digest it. And then, think normally.

Chuck remarked, "Amazes me how Becky faced it with such nonchalance! One would feel the carpet pulled below their feet."

After a few minutes he added, more as if he was making an assessment.

"Such an upheaval would destroy fabric of any family, as hands that hold a family together, were Becky's and they were gone! That's women power... to stand firmly rooted to preserve their families during adversity. If Becky had buckled, her family would be down in the sands."

Each of them in the room felt their hearts miss a beat as they searched their souls. They were left finding deep pools of emotion call it pride or sympathy, or awe in seeing someone larger than life. Becky's brave front left them speechless! They were humbled by her fight to survive and were overcome by respect. In a sudden flash they understood Amy's unquestionable attachment to her new friend. No wonder, the exceptional quality of their mother's friendship, and what had kindled it.

April came and so did Becky's birthday. Amy had made subtle references to Becky of a surprise outing followed by lunch. Everything was planned. Both girls longed for their hour-long chat over a leisure lunch.

Amy was right in anticipating Becky's joy on the special treat that awaited her at the spa. It was all very exciting. Soon some great surprises unfolded, that caught Amy off guard. It started with the gown being handed over for the dress change. Becky whispered to Amy, "Can you please come with me?"

As they moved to the changing-room Amy realized that Becky would need some help. Gradually to prepare for the session, Becky had to remove the prosthetics, before she could finally get upon the table. Amy was struck by the small structure on the table. She smiled willing herself to remain composed.

The attendant came in, dimmed the lights and talked to her prospect enthusiastically, "Becky, let's get you completely relaxed and begin with a hand massage!"

"I have no hands!" Becky stated simply, unflinchingly.

"Oh my-then let's start with your legs," the aesthetician continued changing course.

"I don't have feet!"

Suddenly being made aware that the person on her table had no movable limbs, the attendant burst into tears, rushing out in utter shock. As promised, the Manager hadn't explained Becky's case to her!

Amy patted Becky's arm as she followed the lady into the lobby. Seeing the body shaking emotionally, she spoke soothingly, "Its' okay, you know. No problem. But you must calm yourself. Try and forget this incident and start afresh. It's her birthday so we must make it super special. Give her a facial that she will enjoy. This is her first date at a spa after her accident and she simply loves to get pampered."

With prompting from Amy, the attendant went back and brightened the room with her smile asking for preferences of fragrances, tucking a towel here, raising the bed and making Becky comfortable.

Leaving the duo, Amy slipped out.

Once in the confines of the private space in her car, she started the ignition. She couldn't believe that without her prosthetic legs Becky would be so small. How challenged should Becky feel everyday of her life! By now Amy's body was shaking, sobbing at her own inadequacy for not being to handle her sentiments. Warm tears rolled down her checks in torrents, inconsolable pain wrecking her mind and body. Crying to quell her thumping heart, moaning for her friend's loss, so many years late, in which time Becky had conquered many fears, lived through dark phases when many personal aspirations had gone out crashing.

Amy was very confused. What to think! What to do! She shifted uncomfortably in the car seat, trying to get her thoughts clear, all the while hugging her body to shield it against an unknown fear.

'Poor Becky...no I can't use that word for her. But, God how can she handle so much! We are both so similar! Mother, sister and daughter! But she has so many challenges to handle!'

In a flash some bits of conversation between them came back,

"I found it most difficult to learn to walk again. But using the prosthetic hands was simply impossible."

The agony raised her heartbeat. Becky occupied her thoughts. How many problems' her friend suffered in her every day life.

As she sat huddled behind the wheel, Amy made a decision. She would help her friend in every way she could. Suddenly she felt in control and she walked back to the spa in a happy frame of mind. Over lunch with Becky, she steered the conversation.

Becky mentioned an article she had recently read about a new type of hand transplant that

could restore a recipient a complete control in movement of their fingers. "If I just had a right hand, life would be considerably easier," sighed Becky.

"But it's a kidney transplant that I desperately need. They have me on the national list since 2009 as yet no matching donor has been found. I am a difficult match because of the entire trauma my body has undergone," Becky Springer said unflustered by the way the conversation was going.

After lunch they did some clothes shopping. Becky had weight issues during weekends when she gained 10-15 pounds due to a long gap between dialysis sessions. So with Amy's help Becky tried clothes and bought some loose dresses.

All through the shopping, events of the day and pieces of conversation played on Amy's mind. Next day she called Piedmont

Hospital where Becky was registered and took an appointment with the nephrologist.

It was a few days later when Becky and her nurse were readying for dialysis that Paul came down hesitantly. For convenience and better quality life Becky had changed to peritoneal dialysis. The machine was installed in the basement. "Becky, hospital called. They have a willing, live donor. Your blood needs to be drawn for a tissue match. Identity of the prospect is undisclosed. So we may have a surprise!" His eyes were shining brightly and he even winked at her.

Becky felt a knot forming in her stomach. But as always, her mind ruled over heart enough to recognize it as irrelevant to raise her expectations. She would wait for positive signs. Her thoughts hovered around her life and family. Her three wonderful daughters, Ashley, Mary Catherine and Gretchen!

"How devastated they were when she returned without her limbs. But they quickly assumed additional responsibilities...Ashley took her role as eldest very seriously...but Mary and Gretch were also helpful... God had given me such valuable gems. Oh well we managed, thanks to Paul who was most burdened!"

Her eyes were moist, lips spread in a smile.

"Five years flew by...now Ashley has grown into a young lady... Mary is in her teens and Gretch still almost a kid...hmm!"

Heaving a big sigh she settled down to reality of being dialysed. Few hours later she would be planning the family meal.

Amy was busy with some important meeting when the call came. She took her call and was spellbound to hear that it was a perfect match. But they added that it was highly improbable to have such a perfect match; the test could be wrong. They were scheduling a repeat test soon.

At some point of time Becky became privy to the highly confidential information that it was Amy who had tested and most wonderfully, her tissue match on all six parameters were bang on, with Becky's!

But Amy and Becky faced many trying moments of uncertainty. Doctors were not satisfied that a 100% match was possible! Somehow repeated tests revealed same results! Amy had to follow the protocol process for kidney transplant evaluation. Amy got occupied with the variety of scans, tests, x-rays and ultrasound.

Finally Amy was able to donate the kidney on 3rd June 2011.

Even as Becky's new kidney kicked in, urine forming, her skin changed color from ash, pale yellow to a bright pink. It had a healthy glow and happiness spread around as this dramatic change was noticeable.

Some months later, Becky reflected on how though personally life had changed for her with the kidney transplant Ashley, Mary Catherine and Gretchen had not shown any great enthusiasm. It struck her that kidney helped her lead a normal life as far as diet, passing urine normally and importantly no dialysis. But her girls did not see it bring any change in their lives. If she got back her hands and legs that would be a significant change and bring smiles on their faces.

Yes, she should work towards that.

It was the last week of March 2014. Becky reached out to pick up her new cell phone that beeped aloud.

"Hey Becky" said the warm and friendly voice, one that Becky could recognize even in sleep.

"Oh...Hey Amy...What's up?"

She continued excitedly, "Remember the patch with orchids that I am growing...so they look so amazing!... You must come by...I am watering them as I speak with you."

A few minutes later they spoke of other things, about the family and then Becky could finally say what mattered most to her. "Amy, everyday I think of it. I want to say it now. God sent you to me. We met for a purpose. You came into my life to be the kidney donor with such a perfect match."

"I have no other explanation for our friendship, Amy. Thank you so much for being there for me!"

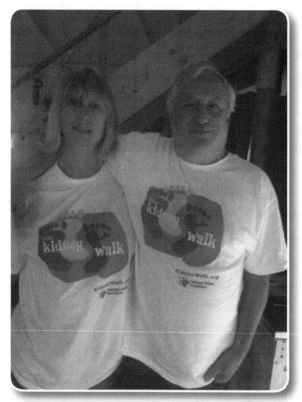
Mark Rosen (Maintenance Treatment) with wife Patti

HIDE AND SEEK WITH CREATININE!

"What does a man do when a sudden stranger knocks at the door?" said Mark, smiling at his friend. "I'm the cancer on your right kidney, is what the stranger said!" he said nonchalantly.

The friend was dumbstruck at first. "What happened Mark?" he asked with disbelief.

Mark said, "Shoo, go away! I barked, quickly got admitted into the hospital. After going through detailed discussions, the right kidney was surgically removed."

Of course Mark knew what it meant removing an organ, but the emotional waves that kept him ravaged was something he had to deal with. His wife Patty proved his greatest supporter, as she bravely held his hand, making it a less harsh reality.

2010 went flying away. Mark opened a fresh diary in January 2011, summoning his strength and self-motivation to move on.

"I'm not letting cancer determine my life. It can't kill my seafarer's spirit, sailing and fishing in Alaska! My love for life in the blue waters; what peace it gives me!"

But Mark grew very sincere in his maintaining a track on his health. On the doctor's advise, he did a battery of tests, wonderingly, yet hoping that it was the last of hospital visits.

Seeing his lab reports, Mark noticed higher levels for creatinine. So the meeting with the nephrologist was going to be not going to be fun! Shaking his head, the nephrologist confirmed he was having an issue with his kidney; he was at stage 4 of the kidney disease.

Mark felt as if the 'Damocles sword' was now hanging just above his head, waiting to axe him anytime. It frightened him to his wits end. Every three months he needed to go and get his tests done. If the kidney function fell below 15%, the doctor said he would need dialysis.

Patty was equally disturbed. It was important to understand what triggered creatinine and proactively, she researched on how to postpone dialysis.

Both Mark and Patty were absolutely clear. Mark should be saved from getting into dialysis by maintaining the kidneys function as presented by this test.

Patty was spot-on when she unraveled the key driver to the disease was diet. If they could nail down the best diet to manage creatinine, they would be saved from great hardships. Armed with this revelation they approached the nephrologist seeking a recommendation for a good, renal dietician.

It took a few weeks for the doctor to direct them to a renal dietician. Somehow the dietician shared very limited information. It gave the couple little confidence to meet the challenge of a life-threatening disease.

"This is so confusing. We are left with nothing, but fear! Such peripheral information for this disease..." Mark spoke out, as soon as he could get out of his shock. "Will I be able to lead a safe life, without dialysis?"

Then he began exploratory work, even when other disturbing thoughts chased his mind. Suddenly a conversation with a friend gave them a clue and a new direction. At first it was difficult to comprehend but research helped..

And voila! Or you can say, it was a Eureka moment.

Mark decided to start a FB page. It began as a learning process, gaining information on kidney disease and renal diet. Slowly people with some stage of kidney disease joined. They would ask questions, to which Mark had a quick reply. It was learning and sharing group as many members shared some great information they had gathered during their rough ride through unknown territories.

Gradually the Facebook group just grew larger and more focused information and discussions happened. The group grew to about 1100 members from world over. Everyone was there to help and support each other.

As the group grew Mark was also making many decisions on his diet and health. From the lab reports he felt he understood the renal diet and also learnt a lot about the disease. On trying to explain his diet, Mark would say he kept mostly the same diet but would cheat sometimes. But within a short time he would bounce back on the proven track. Fortunately it helped him.

His diet was simply tailored to match his lab results. He had to keep all parameters within acceptable levels.

If you were to flip through Mark's diary, this abstract will keep you mesmerized. Mark had recorded his plans; his mental thought process and how through simple tweaking of diet he achieved some good results.

Date eGFR and creatinine	Action plan/ observations
Jan 2011 – 19%	
Aug 2011 – 19% to 32%	Credit: Diet and exercise. Walking 3-7 miles a day. He tells his teammates - "This does take work, but we have to look at what we want in life! For me, it's to be able to live... fish, hunt, or just play with the grand children... I want a productive life. So I continue the fight for health… we can do this together and learn from each other… Just one more thing... I am very proactive with my health… I have my blood work done each month so I know how I am doing...I was also told I have multiple myeloma and that turned out to be okay and then I was told I have lupus and that too is not a problem for me."

09/23/12: GFR down to 21% from 27%	"I do not know what I am doing to make this happen... still eating and exercising.... just more stress and depression set in and now seems to be gone"
12/15/12: eGFR 31.8%; creatinine was 2.1	Blood pressure went up; now normal
01/08/13	Tomorrow I have appointments with Urologist, Oncologist and Nephrologist...a little feeling nervous
01/09/13-eGFR 30%; Creatinine 2.2	
April, 2013 –eGFR down to 26%	
May, 2013 - eGFR-34%	Only change-cut out chicken and turkey from my diet. Now eating only fish...
June, 2013 - eGFR 32% Creatinine 2.0	Dietary changes made. Moved to mostly veggie diet. Fish - 3 times a week. Tough, he felt it would be worth the effort....
Aug. 2013	New nephrologist wants blood work every 3 months. Feel good to be in stage 3... Not stressing as before... Have let go of my past; deal with each moment as it comes...I know for me it is important to stay hydrated, and to eat a healthy renal diet and exercise daily.... but keeping stress down for me is a top priority...

12/30/2013 eGFR of 32	Will be changing my diet again and see if these changes help improve my numbers!
01/10/2014 - eGFR 25%	Doctor testing me for everything scans, blood tests; trying to figure out what is going on...MRI and seeing oncologist in 2 weeks the fun begins again...
02/26/2014 - eGFR was 28%	Try to get back to 30%. "Low white blood cells. Is my multiple myeloma still active?
5/02/2014 eGFR down - 34 to 25%	On 5/7 - 24 hour urine test and blood work... hope to see improvements....
5/17/2014 eGFR is back to the 30% range	Bad news: likely liver problem. Doctor has ordered another lab test for next week
6/26/2014 eGFR back up to 30%	Got a call from my Doctor my liver function is normal... stress, stress and then back to normal
7/01/2014	Given up Face Book. I just did'nt feel I had the ability to help anyone anymore. The stress of the groups daily is upsetting me. I worry about my inability to help heal all... not even able to heal myself...Children with kidney disease is hard for me. Boy I only wish I had a kidney give to them all.
07/15/2014 - eGFR is 39	WOW! Today's results, what a joy!
09/09/2014 eGfr; Creatinine 40 1.72	Thanks to all of you for your help...

10/20/2014 eGFR 41; Creatinine 1.6	Doing better than last month wow this is amazing... so happy...
11/25/2014 eGFR went from 41 down to 38	Okay, what happened? I was dehydrated... will work hard on hydration... am I worried... no, not at all... This is kidney disease; It will have my ups and downs... it can do me much more harm if I start to obsess about all of this... so T-Day is coming... holiday time... family time... just enjoy your time.... Mark Rosen
02/15/2015	Changed my diet...from a raw diet back to cooked... having diarrhea not good... so will see if I can improve with the change.... will be having blood tests on the 18 and then next week appt with Neph... will update after doctor appointment...
2/24/2015 eGFR 41; creatinine is 1.68	Labs keep improving and again I feel it is hydration, diet and exercise and keeping my stress low...
04/02/2015 eGFR is 41; no change creatinine 1.68 - stage 3	Working to reach stage 2, looking into what adjustments I can make to the diet and exercise... is this where it stops? Is this the best it gets for me? Can I reach this new goal of stage 2?

8/12/15 eGFR went from 37 to 40 this time	This is proof to keep stress low in my life… stress messes up my mind and body… great improvement…very happy… all other doctor appointments went pretty well… need to get more tests for liver… thing here is kidney function is improving again…
10/26/2015 eGFR 40	Got home from oncologist all labs very good. Liver is better and cancer number better… I feel good today and thankful for my diet and how I keep improving…
11/23/15 - 2 weeks before eGFR of 40 and now 33%	Big movement… why? Guessing it is the king crab eaten in between blood tests, which I felt gave me the gout… Am I right? But it is a good educated guess… the gout adds stress to the body… anyway will have to pull up my big boy pants and make some major adjustments to diet! Maybe just have to practice more ways to get rid of the stress I give myself…
June 2016 eGFR 36	Doctor appointment today…. wow… it is a progressive disease… eGFR 36, not feeling good about this… going up to 4 Bicarbonate of soda a day now… 650mg will post more later…. this is just the start…
June 2017 all steady but pain in calf muscles	Manganese levels are down… need to improve it…

People like Mark Rosen seem to have a single thought process. *"Keep Kidney Function Tied Down To Same Spot"*. But it was the toughest challenge for him. And he tried to beat it down. It was managed for six years. And with tweaking his diet he continued to fight it down.

Road for kidney patients is tough. But lesser travelled roads will keep you inspired. Keep you wanting more.

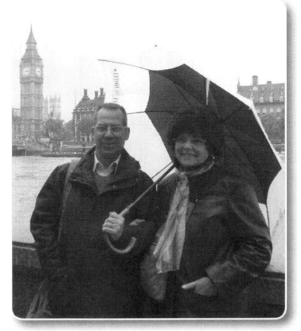

Magda Bonacina (Preemptive Transplantee) and husband Paolo

WAR WAGING WITHIN – MAGDA BONACINA, ITALY

Six-year-old Magda, pulled her scarf tight, closer around the neck, as if guarding something. "Mama asked me to keep the cold morning air away!" she thought, as she looked at the grey, fog-laden sky, making the road to school less visible. Milan was always known to be a cold town, with thick curtains of fog.

The chat and laughter around her drew her attention. She quickened her steps to walk with the girls. As her eyes moved from shoe upwards, she noticed that none of them wore pants; hers' was what in modern times is called a panty hose, which was unheard of in those times, in Italy, as part of women's clothing.

"But…Mama says I should protect myself against cold. I love school. Love walking with them, love their laughter and chatter…. Why worry about my clothes being different? I must not fall ill. I hate to stay at home on school days."

She shrugged away all such random thoughts. "It doesn't matter!"

When her mother, encouraged her to eat meat, "You will keep warm and build resistance against cold and cough." Magda would look into the earnest eyes of her parents, Alma and Luciano and force herself to eat as much as possible. Being frail, she was susceptible to colds. She was fed mostly on meat apart from good nutritious soups. Herbal teas were given to her when she was ill. Much effort was made to keep her well.

What was wrong with Magda?

Was it the polluted environment, from the period of Second World War and after, in Milan?

The Second World War was perhaps the most poignant periods in world history. War about soldiers, conspiracy and calamities, also marked birth of nuclear warfare signifying a mysterious future. Living with terror in their hearts, with stories of violence inscribed in their mind, left them cold. Long drawn warfare, huge loss of lives, created deep wedges in people's hearts, wiping off love for fellow humans.

During the war families living near Milan's military camp, battled with many problems. German forces had taken over Milan, converted the rubber and car engine factories into war weapons manufacturing units. Thick toxic smog turned blue skies to grey, apart from giving many civilians respiratory diseases. Intermittent coughing came to be recognized as tuberculosis, for which treatments were unheard of during that period.

Magda was a two-month-old baby when she contracted a whooping cough. Her parents were anxious and were in fear that it would be tuberculosis. But it turned to be allergic asthma.

Luciano worked in a factory, and later started writing for sports magazine, while Alma became a writer of history books for kids. They were both well-read and worldly wise so they did their own research.

In those days when bronchodilator sprays were not invented, it was very tough to manage Magda's health. Alma wondered if Magda's asthma was a food related allergy. In 1955 little was known of allergies and psychosomatic diseases. However, Alma's persistence helped her find an allergologist whose prescription of a steroid that could cure Magda's asthma, seemed too drastic a treatment and risky. Alma quickly turned down that option for fear of reaching an irreversible condition.

Taking the doctor's other suggestion seriously Alma took Magda to a sea-town, where weather was reasonable. Magda recouped and went back to school a year later.

Waging a war with an invisible enemy was tough, but Alma trudged on. Suddenly it dawned on her. "Am I being obsessed about Magda's health? Should I spend time like a mother with a daughter or only think of her asthma? I always wonder what to do next!"

Soul searching confirmed the bitter truth. Determined as she was, Alma changed her attitude before it became a malady. Suddenly shaking her head she decided, *"Magda should become independent!"*

Magda was sent to spend her vacation with relatives and friends.

Hesitant at first, but in a while Magda began enjoying outings with friends, learnt how to manage her life. It was a new experience being in company of young cousins and friends. They did many wonderful things together. An occasional cough was well managed by her. Time away from home she observed how elders around were carefree. With some guilt she realized how her parents were very concerned about her health.

A period of learning began. Managing health and awareness of what happened around her, seeing people enjoy life, laughed, danced and eat anything at all.

"They are lucky. They have no health worries!" she thought shrugging her shoulder indifferently.

And then Magda met Paolo at one of the mountain vacations. Their friendship grew deep and long lasting. In her final year of schooling, she contracted Hepatitis 'A'. It was some fish consumed by her that brought the infection. Magda spent a year at home to recover. All the time she was aware that Paolo, studying to be a lawyer, was marching ahead. Guilt and determination were triggered so Magda worked hard to complete her education. She consciously put her health in the back burner.

After graduation, she looked back at the rough road she had traversed, through thick fog of toxic air and survived it all. All that seemed well worth as Magda realized with an inward pride, that in spite of frequent tussle with asthma she had made it!

Paolo was her man. They were married when she was 22 years, and lived in Genova, on the Mediterranean coast. Paolo was kept busy in the court as a lawyer, while Magda began teaching at a high school Italian Literature, History, Ancient Latin language. She was also a part-time researcher at Genova University on Medieval Latin manuscripts.

As Magda's father-in-law was discovered with a genetic disease, they chose to adopt a child. Bringing up Michele, schoolwork and family responsibilities kept her busy. But her life's course changed in her 38th year. Suddenly old nightmares broke through their cage threatening her peace and happiness. She came face to face with life's most harrowing moments.

It was a simple fever, with flu-like symptom. But when she found blood in her urine she could feel ground under feet rock her.

"Was this a sign of cancer?" were her first thoughts.

A single episode, but it was enough to freak her out completely. Even as this bizarre thought entered her mind, her mother's early training asked her to unleash her weapon. Find out more. At first the information was overwhelming, but gradually when she realized it was not cancer, she was more relaxed.

Blood in urine was known as "Gross Hematuria." She met doctors and medical experts who were unable to give it any definite prognosis (also if they supposed an IgA nephropathy). It took nearly six years search to arrive at any conclusion. In 1990 a biopsy confirmed it was a Berger's disease, a type of IgA (an autoimmune disease).

A few years later over afternoon tea Paolo and Magda casually started a discussion, which revolved around her IgA research.

Magda explained in a troubled voice, "90% patients get diagnosed only after a casual episode of gross hematuria, because IgA is a silent disease. For some people it may take years for any symptom to surface. Another interesting part of IgA is that it could grow fast into a full-blown disease in some while in others it was less aggressive, which meant slow progression of the disease."

Paolo was amazed at such detailed information and knowledge that she had acquired. Looking into her clear, earnest eyes he said encouragingly, "It means so much work has been done by you. Can you imagine what this information will mean too many people who don't understand the disease?"

"I know, I was lucky and yes, I must share it with people." In the twinkle of her eye he could see he had ignited a purpose. He squeezed her hand encouraging her to go all out, spreading her knowledge.

Magda started with writing a blog. She became a part of IgA groups in Europe, USA and on participated in conferences. She became an advocate for the IgA and became admin on Facebook. Gradually what started as a small, by the side work, she became a full-fledged campaigner for spreading awareness of the disease. As her role grew, she continuously learnt more about IgA.

- It is a genetic autoimmune mediated disorder that affects kidneys, when the genetic anomalies are triggered by some external factors (as infections, vaccines, viruses).
- It is genetic but not directly hereditary, also if it can run in families (especially in Asian families).
- Usually it manifests after an episode of respiratory infection, cough and cold. Apart from the cola –colored urine, a back pain below the ribs, protein in urine, swelling in hands and feet and sometimes, digestive issues.
- IgA's antibodies are generated in respiratory tract mucous and in intestinal mucous.
- IgA's antibodies get deposited into glomeruli gradually, but its' pace of impacting kidney functions was at a slow rate. In most cases it is not aggressive and there is no definitive treatment.

Her own reaction to the episode of hematuria and what she gathered in her research made her draw some definite conclusions:

- Seeing the urine, dark in color makes IgA a disease that generates high-levels of anxiety. Patients faced loneliness and young people became depressed.
- It is best confirmed after a biopsy.
- Life changes, as patients begin to understand and accept that sometime in future the kidneys could be losing its function.

But the real killer was the suspense and unpredictability of the disease.

- As the disease is a recent development, even nephrologists are unsure of its' progress.

No major change was observed in Magda's health. They went on family holydays, she could attend her school and social life was not impaired. But her mind was held captive by her anxiety. Paolo would laugh it away, "Que Sara Sara, whatever will be, will be! If it comes, we will manage it," he said encouraging her.

Now, with 31 years living with IgA, she's able to accept her condition without any qualm. She faced some weakness, but her low hemoglobin has not yet been corrected by an EPO injection, to treat anemia. Maybe in the future, being anemic could be concerning. The creatinine fluctuates between 2.4 and 2.8; proteinuria fluctuates between 250 mg and 350 in 24 hours. Importantly she has maintained the levels for the past 10 years or more.

What did Magda do right?

She was conscious and strict with diet; adopted vegetarian, low protein and low salt diet. She permitted herself an occasional treat with a small serving of meat. Though potassium was not a problem, vegetables were partially leached. Alcohol consumption and cigarette smoking were never tried by her ever, so narcotic drugs were something she didn't dream of. Regular, scheduled blood tests three-six months, diligent about taking medications-for BP, cholesterol, uric acid, calcium, vitamins and folic acid. Additionally as fish oil was suggested as potentially good, Magda took a daily dose.

Early food habits inculcated by her mother, made her choose conservative diet plans, where she left out all packaged food with heavy preservatives and sauces for fear of hidden salt. She included bread, cakes and pasta in her diet along with special renal food that were low in sodium, potassium, phosphorus, low vegetable proteins that incorporated rice, maize and potatoes. She avoided deserts with eggs and cream.

None of these was a renal diet recommended by her doctor.

Now she knows somewhere, at some point in her life, the disease will brush her; it may even decide to live with her and be part of her life. Till then she will try and bring change to many lives.

Her professional growth & knowledge base:

Magda's quest for information never ceases. Every opportunity to expand her portfolio, she grabs and takes it forward. In recent times, it meant formation of a children's group for IgA and HS Purpura.

Facebook groups as admin or co-admin:
Insufficienza renale cronica-IRC (CKD)
Nefropatia Iga/Sindrome di Berger (Gromerulonefrite)
Bambini & insufficienza renale
IgA nephropathy
Renal Patient Support Group
Kidney Disease-Information updates
Kids and Kidney Disease: Not Child's Play
United Children-Kidney desease
Mark's Private Kidney Group Page
The Transplant Community Outreach
Transplantados
Nefropatìa por IgA
Children with IgA nephropathy & HS Purpura

They are 3 Italian, 1 from Argentina, 1 from Spain/Latin America, 1 UK and the others from the USA.

Magda is also editor of some renal magazines (Rein écos; Notizie dal mondo Associativo http://www.emodializzati.it/category/notizie-dal-mondo-associativo/)

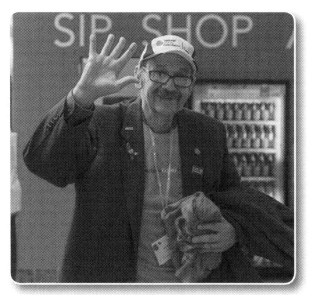

James Myers (Transplantee)

KIDNEY ADVOCACY RULES – JAMES MYERS

Young James grew in a household with lots of mystery.

There was always some whisper down the long corridor. James would be puzzled. *Why were they talking so softly? They don't want me to hear?*

Then he would notice his uncle and his two aunts exchange strange looks that only they seemed to understand. His father would join them sometimes in such conversations. *So what were these secrets?*

As if they realized that James was puzzled they would reach out to pat him briefly and then continue with their chats, looks and nods as if something big was being planned. Somehow he could sense there was some mystery, it was like a blanket of sorrow hanging so heavily that one could barely breathe fresh, clean air in their company.

But his mother was extremely sensitive to his needs. She treated him as a child who needed love. She would make extra efforts to cheer him up with her bright and cheerful chats.

As he grew up, he heard them talk about things like *blood pressure.* James could not make anything out of these discussions. But one day, the words *kidney disease* crept into the conversation along with *BP, creatinine and protein.* Now these became the new buzz-words and James began to follow the conversation with these words without understanding it's significance.

When he questioned his mother she explained to him about how his father, uncle and aunts were all suffering from a very serious kidney disease.

After some thought he asked her, *so do I also have it Mom?*

His mother hushed him, hugging him tightly and asked him to not say such things. The way his mother had explained made James appreciate his family elders and be kind to them.

At times he would look around the house. *Everyone here is pretty sick!*

As he grew he began to feel it was normal for households to have such chats. Young James thought it has been so much part of his life for so many years and yes, nothing abnormal. *But was it similar in other households too?* On some off days James would wonder as he loitered around the corridor as he went off to study. At times he hated it all and at other times he behaved he was above such chats and that none of them bothered him. One thing that struck him was all his family members had this artificial smile painted on their sad faces. This was a façade and they played it always hoping to make him feel better. Seeing them suffer, he would shrug his shoulders.

But the situation changed one day. When James Myers was 25 years old Polycystic Kidney Disease (PKD) became part of his life. It struck him like a thunderbolt and he became aware he had joined the bandwagon of kidney patients in the family.

And then, the scene changed in the family.

His 32 year-old cousin Rich died due to kidney disease. That he was as young as him, made James feel insecure and he was very disturbed. One by one the other diseased elders, except his father, departed. So the house was shrouded in sorrow and pain.

No more were there whispers in the corridors, no more mystery in the air. Now the disease was very much around the house with sorrow and pain in every look of people living in it.

In 1983 his father began dialysis. Dialysis did not seem to go well with his father, who was very uncomfortable and was really troubled by his dialysis sessions. James saw him suffer and this added to his deep hurt and sorrow. Finally his father succumbed to CKD.

James became unsure and wondered: *How will I live through this nightmare of a disease?*

In a quieter moment, with all earnestness James decided to take a control of his health. He made many lifestyle changes, which seemed as big sacrifices. But ignoring those pangs of temptations James managed to remain well for 34 years.

But things changed slowly and he could sense that his control was slipping. Small signs showed up which was confirmed by the doctor to be bad signs.

"Jim, I think it's time to start your real treatment." The physician said with a little nod, lips pursed, eyes showing regret.

Preparation work for fistula began making James very unhappy with the situation he had landed himself in. But he realised how important dialysis was for his health. So he settled down his dialysis schedule. But he also made time to register on 3 transplant lists. He needed a transplant. He constantly wondered, *When will I ever eat a slice of chocolate cake, with no guilt attached? How I long for a hassle free future without worrying about my kidney disease, simply enjoying life as it flowed with eat a complete meal without any restriction.*

Rolling his eyes, smacking his lips he laughed at the mere thought of that joyous moment.

One day at the dialysis center a friend was curious on how James had managed to remain away from dialysis for so long.

"Ah!" James said thoughtfully.

"I just followed all the rules of the game. My physician told me to reduce a portion of my protein intake, add less salt in my food and eat healthy meals with salad and fruits. So that was my diet."

Mulling over how he lived the past few years James continued, "I made regular visits to Indiana University Kidney Clinic to make sure my blood pressure was under control. I never missed medications. So BP meds and diet were things I never lost sight of. Very strict with these two buddies all my years."

The friend rolled his eyes and said, "If only I knew dialysis could be postponed. I feel ashamed for being irregular with tests and medicines."

Another friend who had joined into the conversation asked James, "Jim, were you also working during this period?"

"Indeed, I was working as a trial lawyer, but eventually I couldn't be active so stopped working. But I was very lucky on two counts. I could work as a college professor and delay dialysis for so long."

One day it occurred to him this genetic condition could also affect the future generations. He spoke to his son, "Son, I need you to go through some tests as Polycystic Kidney Disease has already been with us for two generations... let's see if you're inheriting it as well."

It was the happiest day for James when his son PKD tests were negative.

"Thank God we beat it!" he said, most thankfully.

James spent a few years on dialysis and every day he posted seeking for a live kidney donor.

By April 2016, all his pre-transplantation tests were completed. Finally James got "the call".

A lady spoke, ""Hi, may I speak with James Myers?" "Yes, it's me!" That voice grew excited and said those magical words "We have a kidney for you!"

James got his kidney and he christened him "Woody Woodrow." the

> All his life being intensely made aware of the kidney disease and fighting it for so many years, he got worked up when he realised that while incidence of kidney disease was rising, not much awareness was there about the disease. Many people could have been saved with early detection if they managed their blood pressure and diabetes. Polycystic Kidney disease was a genetic disease so unavoidable but progression could be slowed, which was also possible for diabetes and hypertension.
>
> James joined Facebook and opened several groups.

There along with many others he would share important information and slowly advocacy work began. But he had much bigger contribution coming his way.

James shared with us how deeply he was aggrieved.

"When I was on dialysis, a law to cut funding to all dialysis centers was being proposed. It made me very angry. I looked around the room. All my clinic mates were too sick to fight back. I was the only one who had the energy in me, along with a strong sense of righteousness to stop this law that could terminate many lives. So I acted.

I joined several national organizations, including the National Kidney Foundation. I wrote several petitions and opinion against editorials. I visited Members of Congress in Washington, DC. I started to be more active online. Eventually, the law was defeated. I have been a kidney advocate ever since".

In 2015, James was honored with the National Social Media and Advocacy Award from the American Association of Kidney Patients. In the NKF, he is now the Statewide Advocate for the State of Indiana. James is a member of an elite group of advocates, the Kidney Advocacy Committee. He is a Regional Leader for Region #5 in the USA, consisting of the States of Michigan, Ohio, Indiana, Kentucky & Tennessee. He meets advocates from those states to give advice and support."

James Myers is now waiting to go back to teaching. It was all about connecting with people with a story to tell.

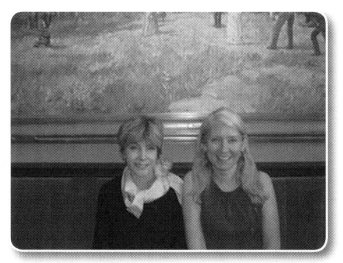

Sally Satel (Transplantee) and Virginia Postrel (Altruistic Donor)

ISN'T IT HIGH TIME TO REVIEW?
– SALLY SATEL AND VIRGINIA POSTREL

I always felt asking for a kidney was most difficult. But as I looked around, I found altruistic kidney donors were gaining popularity in the US. Something that should also happen in other countries!

One case that really turned me on was Sally Satel's story. The donor was Virginia Postrel, a renowned author and activist.

In November 2005 Virginia responded to Sally-"Serious offer" as the heading of the mail that read, "If I'm compatible, I'll be a donor. Best, Virginia".

She followed it two weeks later, "By the way, I absolutely promise you that I will not back out".

On 7th March 2006, Virginia returned from the hospital after surgically transplanting the kidney and feeling satisfied. Read on for one of the most remarkable stories in organ donation.

49 year-old Sally Satel, a psychiatrist and lecturer at the Yale University School of Medicine, resident scholar at the American Enterprise Institute was diagnosed with failing kidneys in August 2004. Possibly it meant she could start dialysis six months down the line. No lifestyle condition like blood pressure or diabetes was evidenced for onset of the disease. Nephrologists believed it could be due to some medication taken nearly thirty years ago. It was an idiopathic kidney failure, which was a kind of *glomerular disease.*

She got herself listed at the national organ transplant listing at number 61,000 at that time.

She did some investigation, studied data and realized that it could well be over five years before she would be allotted a kidney for the transplant. She was not so comfortable with the thought of dialysis, which would alienate her from friends apart from the debilitating effects of the treatment. She had known of patients on dialysis facing experiences-of cramps, vomiting spells and their confinement at home.

Talking to friends, networking on the web for a donor brought some positive results. Two friends almost handed over the kidney; some others tested and were not a good match. Seeking other avenues also meant registering on the MatchingDonors. com. Result emerged with a 62 year old retired Canadian man, responding to her request. Sally was tentative at times, making him comfortable with his offer and they developed a rapport. His earnestness to be the donor became evident when he went into great lengths discussing logistics including the insurance coverage, where and how to transplant the organ. All through there was active conversation during the fall, with a promised 'organ'.

Through a mutual friend, Virginia had heard about Sally Satel looking for a kidney donor. Few years ago they had shared professional interaction on a project. So Virginia sent a mail offer. The Canadian's offer being still 'hot' meant an option for a donor was being pursued.

Sally had seen two friends move away on some pretext, but when shutters went down on the Canadian's offer she was disheartened. Fortunately, Virginia's mail was comforting and gave her hope for relief. Virginia's mails exhibited her intention to behave as a responsible donor, with firm purpose to deliver.

Virginia went through the donor evaluation and took the tests.

She got approved as a donor and the surgery took place.

Reflections:

Why was Virginia Postrel so willing to part with an organ?

Virginia being "brazenly pragmatic" shared her take on donating a kidney, "I have a very instrumental view of my body, so when you needed a part, I was happy to give it".

Virginia felt empathy and realized that since Sally had no family-parents were dead and she had no sibling-she should help her constructively. It was this sentiment aroused in a person momentously that shows us how some people's generosity can peak so high. Some hearts are simply made to be more caring!

To the world this story is unique.

There is no reasoning for Virginia's heart-warming gesture but in Hindu philosophy it comes under the umbrella of what is popularly called "Karma".

But the post transplant scene opened a new thinking.

Surprisingly on this topic both Sally and Virginia were on same line of thinking. For a kidney donor the aura of heroism wanes as soon the economies of the episode surfaces. Bills for travel, stay and additionally loss of pay, punctures the sheer joy of giving when financial reality surfaces. Kidney donors were not getting recognized for sacrifices they made nor did their heroic act gave any great impetus to organ donation.

Sally Satel has been fortunate to have two friends donating a kidney, one in 2006 and the second in 2016. The first transplant "galvanized me about the issue, not the surgery, but the process of finding a donor," she said at one occasion. This deep-seated anguish for humanity, at a vastly different level than commonly viewed, made her vocal about kidney transplants with a new approach.

She analysed the situation in the US:

- Out of 120,000 all organs, 98000 waited for a kidney transplant. Majority of them would wait for a deceased donor.
- "12 people will die tomorrow, by this time," she said because they can't survive the wait. Everyday 12 people on the list will leave. It is indeterminate who will leave first because their end will be determined by individual health condition, mental acceptance and tolerance of dialysis regime!
- In 1984 National organ transplant act defined that altruistic as the sole motivation for giving a kidney. If anyone accepted valuable consideration, they could actually be prosecuted for felony-$50000 and/ or 5 years of imprisonment.
- Many ways were consciously developed to increase the donor pool. Education to sign up for organ donation, special arrangements for emergency rooms to counsel families to release organs of their beloved and such others.
- Swap transplants was meant to be a great game-changer. It was indeed an excellent concept. But sadly the swap gave only 500 new organs - against a requirement from 98,000 individuals!

Kidney

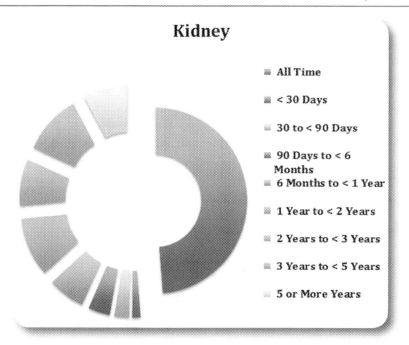

- All Time
- < 30 Days
- 30 to < 90 Days
- 90 Days to < 6 Months
- 6 Months to < 1 Year
- 1 Year to < 2 Years
- 2 Years to < 3 Years
- 3 Years to < 5 Years
- 5 or More Years

Chart developed by Vasundhara

In her view, the ban on financial compensation is an obstacle for organ donation. While she categorically states she doesn't advocate "classic free market" she urges lawmakers to think of ways to incentivize people. A general idea, outline of a model to reward people who help a stranger she suggests could be:

- Tax forgiveness for expenses incurred for organ donation
- Tax credit
- Contribution retirement account
- Children's education voucher
- Loan forgiveness
- Donation to a charity of their choice
- Consideration valued at about $50000 that could come out dialysis savings
- After from safeguarding dignity issues, there won't be any question of exploiting people from low-income group!
- If can follow the first come, first served principle and take the normal time as in other transplants, that's about

3 months – enough time for a donor to get a chance to understand the surgery and its implications and the authorities to check if the person has been coerced.

Elaborating the ground for reviewing the existing system she put together some great observations that is reproduced below:

"Our current transplant regime is a qualified failure. Transplant operations have been basically flat for the last eight years. In 2013, over 4300 people died while waiting and about 3000 were permanently removed from the queue because they developed a medical condition that precluded transplant. Twenty-seven years ago, the average wait for a deceased-donor kidney in the United States was about one year; now, the average wait is approaching five years. In many parts of the country it has reached a ten-year wait from listing to transplant—if one can survive that long."

Further she brings to memory strong words in support of compensations.

But will this proposition find favor amongst people with different outlook? It needs a lesson in humanity and understanding the deep-rooted pain associated with chronic kidney disease.

"And, at one of the early NOTA hearings in the House, Al Gore, then the Tennessee congressman spearheading the legislation, spoke approvingly of "the provision of incentives, such as a [presumably third-party] voucher system or a tax credit to a donor's estate" if "efforts to improve voluntary donation are unsuccessful."

But in the interests of people, struggling every other day to prepare mentally and physically for a session of dialysis, some drastic steps are much needed. Failure to react will wipe out kidney communities as each year more people get recruited.

References: 33 27. See RESTATEMENT (SECOND) OF CONTRACTS § 71(1) (1979)

STATE ORGAN-DONATION INCENTIVES
UNDER THE NATIONAL ORGAN
TRANSPLANT ACT

SALLY SATEL* JOSHUA C. MORRISON** RICK K. JONES***

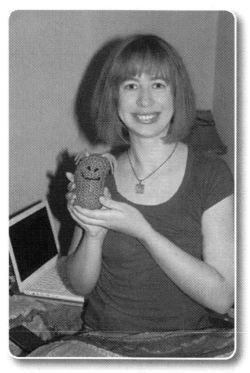

Jenna Franks

KIDNEYS FIND THEIR OWN DESTINATION – JENNA FRANKS

Karol was reminiscing the long journey with kidneys for Jenna over the morning coffee.

It was about small incidents that connected magically to help Jenna on two different occasions. The first incident in 2006 was still quite fresh in sensitivity. She was at her desk when she picked up the phone and the caller began, "Hi… I'm seeking some urgent information on cross match and antibodies…"

Karol was quick to pick up the cause for tension and explained how important it was to have lower level of antibodies so there's no risk to the transplanted kidney. During the conversation she had suggested to the caller, Patrice Smith, to check on other prospects on the "Living Donor's" waiting list.

Patrice gained her composure and went ahead to check the online donor website.

What happened thereafter was a matter of pure coincidence. Patrice actually chose Jenna, Karol's 21-year-old daughter who was also looking for a kidney donor!

The transplant happened much to the joy of the family.

But life of that kidney was limited. Seven years.

The second trip down the "organ search" lane had begun. Today, Karol could sigh as this chapter had come to a close but the days, months and years that built up had many moments that were indelible.

Then an email from Jenna's Godmother had been very comforting.

That day it had played on Karol's mind as she carried through her work. At the dinner table, she had mentioned it. "Oh… by the way, today I had this amazing news from Rhonda. A few days ago, she had posted Jenna's story on her timeline and her friend Gary Frey, a Marine veteran from Tucson had agreed to get tested for Jenna. He's offering her his kidney!"

"That's good news!" her husband Ed said eagerly. Though the news created some buzz around the table, with Jenna, James, Becca and Johnny talking excitedly, Karol added tentatively, "But we need to do the tests before jumping into any conclusions."

Though the topic was put to rest there was some renewed hope for Jenna. For a second transplant she needed a good live donor match. The previous transplant's rejection had left Jenna with very high level of antibodies, making it very difficult to find a match.

Statistically out of 10,000 only 3 people could be her perfect match. So what was the probability that Gary Frey was one of the three!

String of mails from Rhonda and Gary kept the topic 'hot' enough for them to pursue and get the tests done. To have a dialogue with a willing donor was really so blessed as many people on Facebook were looking for a donor.

In a few weeks however, it was confirmed. Gary was a good candidate, but not a match for Jenna.

Over the years many friends, family members and strangers tested, with no success.

But Jenna was not one to keep quiet. Together, she and Gary joined a kidney paired donation program called the National Kidney Registry, a transplant option for prospective recipients who had a willing but incompatible donor. The only way for Gary to donate to a recipient was for there must be a suitable match for Jenna, but no match had been found since registering for the program.

Surprisingly Gary stayed committed for five years.

Finally the big day arrived. Gary's kidney got transplanted on 18th July 2017.

With Gary giving away his kidney, the transplant team at UCLA began working on Jenna's antibodies with treatments of Rituximab, plasmapheresis, thymoglobulin and IVIG. Wait and watch game for the right match began.

This period was spiked with worry, planning, with high riding faith that "good luck" would knock at Jenna's door soon. There was a huge suspense built around the timing when the donor would show up. Things were still not completely under her control. Jenna went through each day with great expectations. Hopefully an organ would be found.

And… Hurray…. The moment arrived. In Karol's words, "Call it coincidence or fate, or thanks to Gary's good karma, Jenna got a call from the UCLA transplant team, saying that the National Kidney Registry had found a compatible match for Jenna!"

Being a swap donor, not many details were there! But the joy of it being Jenna's first call in 5 years was heart-warming.

Jenna started desensitization treatments. They showed considerable decrease in her "very high antibodies".

On July 26, 2017, a kidney from an anonymous donor was flown from the North East US to Los Angeles, and Jenna had her transplant surgery. Through the surgery the messages were on social media, there were updates and lots of kind enquiries to be responded. Lots of wishes and prayers came pouring in, so the family was truly overwhelmed.

Karol recalled the few quiet moments in the hospital.

She had looked at her 31-year-old daughter Jenna as she was recovering! What a tough time it had been for Jenna since her high school days. The initial shock that she and the family felt when she was detected with a rare urological defect that silently destroyed her kidneys. Karol thought of how inconvenient it could have been, when there were young girls and boys having a great time. Even while in high school, Jenna had been on dialysis. For three years she had continued on this treatment.

Then phenomenal things had happened.

Karol felt her heart fill with gratitude that in 2012, Rhonda had posted about Jenna needing a donor, and Gary decided to commit to donate.

Karol wondered what made a man wait so long and never considered going back on his promise. It spoke a lot of humanity and singular purpose to do an altruistic act. In her heart the love and respect rose to its' peak for Gary who entered their lives and left a huge treasure. One that was priceless.

Jenna's treatments-plasmapheresis, IVIG and antithymocyte globulin will continue over time, to reduce antibodies to protect her from rejection. She will be on immunosuppressives for life of the transplanted kidney.

The aspect of uncovered expenses for the donor has been a problem in live-donor transplants. A donor's medical expenses are basically covered by insurance, but the donor needs to meet expenses on travel, lodging, and lost wages for time taken off for testing, surgery, and recovery. Federal law prohibits the sale of an organ, but an exception is allowed for "reasonable payments" for those expenses incurred by a living kidney donor. A gofundme campaign was started in this case.

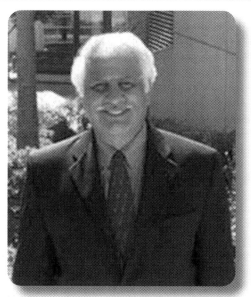

Mohammad Akmal

SELF-DIAGNOSING MY KIDNEY CANCER
– MOHAMMAD AKMAL

It is very normal for me to wake up sometime in between sleep to visit the toilet. But two years ago I had a shocking experience. At 2am even though my eyes were heavy with sleep I noticed flank blood in my urine. The nephrologist in me was fully awake and raised questions, "No pain in the kidney, so is it what I suspect?" I went back to bed and shared my new worry with my wife, "I think I may havea kidney cancer!"

She stirred in bed and responded in a sleepy voice, " What makes you make this comment at this unearthly hour?"

"I just passed blood in the urine and I have no pain. Painless hematuria suggests that it could be kidney cancer!"

I visited my physician next morning requesting for an ultra sound of the kidneys. It showed some swelling of the ureter (left hydroureter). I made a quick mental note, "I must get to the bottom of this!" but with a medical conference in New York I was busy the whole week. Another episode of bloody urine while returning to California became a cause for worry and eventually I decided to focus on my health. Visiting a local hospital in the Bay Area I managed to get an abdomen CT scan done. It revealed a left hydroureter with a tumor that was more than 3 cms in size. Years' of experience helped me conclude that it was transitional cell carcinoma. But I knew it had to be backed with a biopsy.

I headed to an urologist for a biopsy unfortunately he couldn't accomplish the task, as it was difficult to pass the stent to reach the tumor. So the biopsy was halted. When finally the biopsy of the tumor was managed, the diagnosis was confirmed as transitional cell carcinoma. A team of urologists recommended removal of the left kidney, left ureter and evaluate the pelvis area of the urinary bladder.

Before my surgery I underwent another round of tests including a CT scan, MRI and PET scan and the relevant blood tests. These tests showed that the disease was limited to the ureter though some insignificant activity was seen in the pelvis.

A robotic surgery that lasted 14 hours was performed to remove the affected kidney and left ureter. It was longer than usual because of adhesions from previous surgery. After a successful surgery I was discharged after about 5 days stay at the hospital. My postoperative course was excellent.

A few months later, my first surveillance was uneventful. My surgeon congratulated me saying, "It is one of the rare occasions that I can tell the patient you are cured from this cancer."

I can sadly say, cancer is like a chameleon and it can fool us at any time. It resurfaced a few months later putting me on a tough road of recovery.

My second diagnostic imaging showed a new lesion in the previously located kidney area. I approached a general surgeon requesting him to remove the lesion by an open abdominal surgery. In a pre surgery evaluation, some glands were detected in my left neck. Suspecting it to be a second cancer an ultrasound of my neck was done followed by a biopsy of the glands. The tests confirmed it was cancer and so the line of treatment changed.

I was subjected to powerful chemotherapy that I didn't tolerate well. I felt these 6 months of life was my most miserable period in life, as I needed to handle so many complications. Such as the frequent nausea and vomiting episodes, irritation caused by lack of appetite, generalized skin rash, peripheral neuropathy (dead feeling and numbness), weakness of muscles, fatigue, frequent falls and most annoying aspect was my disturbed sleep.

But suddenly some good fortune came my way. During this period immunotherapy was approved in the USA for treatment and many people benefited from it. Doctors were kind enough to offer me immunotherapy, which was intravenously administered once in every 3 weeks. As soon as immunotherapy was initiated, my life miraculously changed. My cancer gradually seemed to be under control. I feel so grateful to God that I was given a second chance to live.

Today I'm able to laugh it away, but there are times when I sit and reflect on what had transpired. It is ironic how a nephrologist who treated so many patients, faced some kind of kidney disease. I also think of how each of my patients' would have faced their life challenging experiences. Now I feel I am in a better position to treat patients by fully appreciating their feelings as I am on their side of the fence.

PART II: MEDICAL FACTS AND EMOTIONAL SUPPORT

Our purpose of adding some pertinent information on medical aspects of the disease is to offer guidance and information. Some disease information was already shared in story narrations but more detailed information of an experienced nephrologist will be found in this section. For more in-depth information you may like to read nephrology journals and other medical books.

This section deals with:

- *Many conditions that could lead to kidney failure – Dr M Akmal*
- *CKD Management, issues and treatments – Dr M Akmal*
- *Safe Pregnancy, for patient and unborn – Dr M Akmal*
- *Patient Centric Aspects: Trauma and need for support - Vasundhara*
- *The ride beyond rejection! – Vasundhara Raghavan*
- *Facing a Kidney Failure – Vasundhara Raghavan*
- *Common glossary terms (Centers for Disease Control and Prevention)*

Thank you.

Dr Mohammad Akmal
Vasundhara Raghavan

MANY CONDITIONS THAT COULD LEAD TO KIDNEY FAILURE

Diabetes and hypertension are recognized as two most common secondary reasons for kidney failure. Kidney failure is related to such pre-existing conditions.

Taking guard

It is established and recognized worldwide that since both diabetes and hypertension could end into a kidney failure, early preventive action is extremely advisable to prevent it to lead into a kidney failure. Periodic blood tests and blood pressure coupled with controlling diet and regular exercise will change the way the future will pan out for patients with diabetes and blood pressure.

Diabetes, with relevance to kidney failure

In my association with patients there were many who courageously met the new challenge of life, which need special mention. But it would be useful to briefly discuss the diabetic associated kidney disease.

Diabetes is a condition when the patient has elevated blood sugar level either because the body does not produce sufficient insulin or the body cells do not respond to the insulin. Insulin, the hormone produced by the pancreas enables the body cells to absorb glucose to turn it in to energy. The definition of diabetes mellitus was recently modified by American Diabetes Association to include several independent criteria to establish the diagnosis such as a 75-g oral glucose tolerance test with a 2-h value of 200 mg/dl, or more, a random plasma of glucose of 200 mg/dl, or more with typical symptoms of diabetes and a fasting glucose of 126 mg/dl or greater on more than one occasions. Fasting glucose values are preferred for their convenience and reproducibility. There are many types of diabetes, the most common of which are:

Type 1: Failure of body to produce insulin

Type 2: Cells fail to use insulin properly, sometimes combined with an insulin deficiency

Gestational: When pregnant woman who never had diabetes before, develops high blood glucose levels during pregnancy. It may eventually result in type 2-diabetes.

As of 2000 at least 171 million people worldwide suffer from diabetes, 2.8% of the population. Its incidence is increasing rapidly, and the number is estimated to double by 2030. [Recent estimates provided by the International Diabetes Federation, Brussels, Belgium gives an estimate of 250 million as of November 2008. Unless deliberate measures are taken by 2030 the incidence will be much higher].

In 2008 the number of diabetics in USA was 24 million; of those 5.7 million remain undiagnosed. Other 57 million individuals are estimated to be pre-diabetic, and an additional 30-40 million people are believed to have impaired glucose tolerance resulting in health care costs exceeding 100 billion dollars annually. Of the two types, type 2 affects 90-95% and 5-10% of the US diabetic population belongs to type 1.

The prevalence of diabetes increases with age. This is supported by real estimates that show 18.3% (8.6 million) of Americans above 60 years are diabetics. Approximately 20-30% of diabetics will develop a kidney disease and about half of the patients who started dialysis are diabetics (a greater percentage with type 2 which has a higher base).

Type-2 diabetes is more common in Native Americans, Hispanics, African Americans, Asians and pacific islanders compared to the Caucasians. The increased incidence in developing countries is partly due to increased urbanization and adopting western life style, particularly on diet. Another emerging group is the youth facing obesity, hence more prone to develop the disease. Besides being potential diabetics, other contributory factors such as high blood pressure, poor control of diabetes, focal segmental glomerulonephritis, lipid abnormalities and smoking puts this age group at higher risk of developing CKD.

Diabetics with CKD carry poor prognosis as those on dialysis or recipients of kidney transplant are faced with increased morbidity and mortality due to coexistent diabetic complications. The poor vision, heart problem, circulatory insufficiency, nerve damage and amputations are additional problems contributing to misery of these patients. Reports show that more than half of the patients die within two years of initiating dialysis.

How will a person know that he is a diabetic?

A person will experience some/one of the following symptoms. Once it is noticed the person can seek doctor's help and necessary medications can be taken to control diabetics.

- blurred vision
- frequent urination
- increased thirst
- weight loss
- slow healing sores
- feelings of hunger and tiredness

Diabetes is a long term disease, which has no cure but with careful control of blood sugar, complications of the disease can be prevented or delayed. However, many people have no signs of the symptoms, before it is diagnosed.

Hypertension

Hypertension, a common chronic medical condition, follows diabetes as the second common cause for CKD. In the 6th century BC the writings of Sushtruta Samhita [a Sanskrit redaction on ayurvedic concepts] were the first to mention symptoms like those of hypertension. The modern understanding of hypertension began with the work of physician William Harvey (1578-1657) and a century later Richard Bright recognized it as a disease entity. Frederick Mahomed was the first to report high blood pressure in a patient without kidney disease (1849-1884).

Locating reason for high blood pressure

As part of its function the heart pumps blood into arteries, which carries blood to all parts of the body. Blood pressure is the measured force of the blood as it hits the walls of the arteries, which is 120 (systolic reading) when the heart pumps and is 80 (diastolic reading) when the heart rests. This is observed in the normal course.

According to the National Heart, Lung, and Blood Institute, (NHLBI) High Blood Pressure (HBP) is a reading of blood pressure of 140/90 mmHg or higher. Both the numbers forming the range are important for assessment of blood pressure. Once a person develops HBP, it generally lasts a lifetime.

Hypertension is classified either as 'essential' (no known medical cause) or 'secondary' (due to another cause, like kidney disease, renal artery stenosis, adrenal tumor, pheochromocytoma, or any other causes).

A recent classification brings clarity to the condition:

Classification	Systolic BP	Diastolic BP
Normal	90-119 mmHg	60-79 mmHg
Prehypertension	120-139	80-89
Stage 1	140-159	90-99
Stage 2	>160	>100
Isolated Systolic HTN	>140	<90

An adult will be known as hypertensive if his BP is high on two or more BP readings, obtained more than one minute apart at two or more visits. *[Note that BP after smoking, eating, and consuming caffeinated beverages will be elevated. So the BP must be measured after an hour of such activity, particularly with salty foods]*.

Physicians specializing in hypertension conduct 24 hour ambulatory BP monitoring before establishing the case as hypertension. Under this monitoring multiple BP readings over a prolonged period of time is obtained. Complete understanding of the condition is possible if the collected information is assessed by these parameters:

- mean 24 hour BP
- mean day time BP
- mean nighttime BP
- average difference between waking and sleeping BP
- evaluates nocturnal dipping (a decrease in mean arterial BP of > 10% during sleep)
- above others variations in BP

As in adults, blood pressure in children is variable between individuals, within individuals, by day and at different times of the day. Study shows distribution of patients with hypertension as:

- Preadolescents: 60-70% is of secondary type and renal parenchymal disease
- Adolescents: 80-90% are largely the essential type
- Adults: 90-95% is the essential type. Among secondary hypertension it is known that primary hyperaldosteronism is the most frequent endocrine form. Hypertension is frequently part of metabolic "X Syndrome" which also includes diabetes, dyslipidemia, and central obesity.

Blood Pressure (BP) is usually measured with a *sphygmomanometer* during a visit to the doctor, though sometimes it maybe done at home by patients. The device derives its name derived from the Greek word 'sphygmós' which means pulse combined with a scientific term for pressure meter, 'manometer'.

Knowing the condition

More than 90% BP patients are with "essential hypertension" while balance 10% cases are with "secondary hypertension". These are how the patients are evaluated in the primary care setting.

"Essential hypertension" is heterogeneous and polygenic condition, resulting from dysregulation of hormones, proteins, and neurogenic factors involved in BP regulation. Dietary factors and inactivity largely contribute towards increase in incidence. Impaired loss of salt by the kidneys plays a pivotal role in the pathogenesis of hypertension. Although 30% to 60% of BP variability is inherited, the common gene that significantly affects BP is yet to be identified.

Polyporphism in alleles at many different loci interact with behavioral and environmental factors resulting in final disease trait. Rare monogenic forms of hypertension have also been identified. Nearly all genes identified playing a role in the pathogenesis of the hypertension cause changes in salt handling by the kidneys, thus providing credence to the importance of excretion of sodium by the kidneys in the development of hypertension.

"Secondary hypertension" is most commonly caused by kidney disease, primary hyperaldosteronism, renovascular disease, and pheochromocytoma.

Other causes include endocrine dysfunction or exogenous factors like oral contraceptives, non-steroidal anti-inflammatory drugs (NSAIDs), erythropoietin (used to correct anemia in patients with renal failure and cancer), calcineurin inhibitors (e.g., cyclosporine and prograf) used for organ transplantation, and sympathomimetic agents (catecholamines, epinephrine, norepinephrine and dopamine).

Patients who have atypical clinical features and are resistant* to therapy for BP control may be considered as those with secondary hypertension. This should be the guiding factor for adopting the line of treatment.

Narrowing hypertension 'type' for treatment

Apart from essential and secondary, further types should be identified and determined. Understanding and elimination of these types will bring clarity for treating the condition.

*Resistant hypertension is characterized by failure to achieve a target BP control with optimal dosages of three medications of different classes of BP medications including a diuretic. There is difficulty in determining if a person is resistant. If a person is non compliant with medications, leading to poor control, it would be wrong to conclude that the person is resistant to therapy when the therapy has been inadequate.

The predisposing factors associated with resistant hypertension include:

- older age
- black ethnicity
- obesity (BMI > 30),
- diabetes underlying hypertension
- medications that may increase BP (cocaine, NSAIDs, cyclosporine, and erythropoietin etc), excessive alcohol consumption and increased intake of sodium.

Before concluding that the person is resistant factors like obesity, sleep apnea, and secondary types of hypertension (primary aldosteronism and renovascular hypertension) should be considered and ruled out.

About 50-60% patients with sleep apnea are affected with hypertension and conversely about 50% of patients with hypertension have sleep apnea. Strong association is particularly found in patients with resistant hypertension and usually results from excessive salt intake, nocturnal hypoxemia-mediated sustained elevated sympathetic nervous system activity, excessive aldosteronisn, and obesity associated insulin resistance.

Some smaller percentage of cases may be found to be "White coat hypertension", "Masked Hypertension" or "Exercise induced Hypertension".

People who are noticed with high blood pressure in the doctor's office are said to have "white coat hypertension". This kind of hypertension is defined by BP measurements above 140/90 mmHg at least during three separate visit at the doctor's office and with at least two sets of measurements below 140/90 mmHg in non clinic settings, in the absence of target organ damage. Some people experience "lab coat syndrome" defined by skyrocketing BP when approached by a medical professional wearing the stethoscope.

The ambulatory BP measurement is considered the gold standard for detecting patients who are 'resistant hypertension' and differentiate them from those with 'white coat hypertension'. This involves checking BP regularly; taking readings at home and/or at work to estimate the average BP measurements in day-to-day real life situations.

Patients with white coat hypertension have a lower risk for cardiovascular disease when compared to those with sustained hypertension. Though these patients have greater tendency to develop sustained hypertension, pharmacologic treatment of white coat hypertension has not shown decrease morbidity.

Masked hypertension is characterized by a normal office BP but high ambulatory BP measurement. This appears to affect about 10 million people in US and definitely carries higher risk for cardiovascular disease when compared to those with normal office and ambulatory BP measurements. Treatment may begin if ambulatory BP measurements are elevated but there are no clinical trials available regarding the treatment of masked hypertension.

Exercise induced hypertension is characterized by the presence of systolic BP of at least 186 mmHg in African American men, 182 mmHg in white men, 174 mmHg in African woman and 162 mmHg in white woman. The upper normal systolic values during exercise reach levels between 200-230 mmHg. The prevalence of left ventricular hypertrophy in these patients is 33% compared to others. Among these patients the prevalence of a low ankle-brachial index is about 40% compared to 18% in others. People with exercise hypertension may demonstrate greater amounts of carotid plaques and a larger left ventricular mass but do not show abnormalities in the exercise ECG or thallium scan. These people appear to have an increased risk of peripheral vascular disease, carotid disease and left ventricular hypertrophy, and exercise hypertension may be a precursor marker of significant vascular disease. The persons with exercise-induced hypertension should be aggressively treated with aggressive cardiovascular risk reduction therapy that should include measures to reduce lipids and blood pressure.

Manage and treat hypertension

Management of hypertension includes lifestyle modifications and drug treatment for all patients with stage 1 or greater hypertension. The goal should be to decrease BP below 140/90 mmHg that is universally applicable for all hypertension patients.

Lifestyle modifications include weight reduction, DASH diet (rich fruits, vegetables, and low-fat dairy products with a reduced content of saturated and total fat), reduction of sodium intake below 2.4 g/ 24 hours, aerobic physical activity for 30-34 minutes most days, and limited daily alcohol consumption to two drinks for men and one drink for women.

If single agent antihypertensive therapy is not effective in 1-3 months of treatment, the consulting doctor should be informed. Change in medication or adding a drug with a complementary mechanism of action may be advised.

Resistant hypertension should be managed by lifestyle modifications stopping the medications that may increase BP, and correction of the secondary causes. Resistant hypertension is usually associated with volume expansion and requires diuretic therapy.

Patients with sleep apnea should receive appropriate treatment with continuous positive airway pressure (CPAP).

In all cases of secondary hypertension, the cause should be identified and treated aggressively.

Generally, it is hard to establish whether kidney failure is due to high BP or due to a kidney disease. However, essential hypertension is responsible for more than 90% of cases and a good history, nature of previous follow up and appropriate diagnostic evaluation may help in the establishing the correct diagnosis.

Finally, hypertension is predominantly from an unknown cause. It is prudent to rule out secondary causes because treatment of some of these conditions may provide a permanent cure of hypertension. Unfortunately, inadequate measures in diagnosis of hypertension and its poor control result in enormous human, economic and medical costs to the society.

Combination with diabetes

In patients with diabetes, hypertension adds significantly to the risk of vascular disease and death. It is recommended that hypertension in these patients should be aggressively controlled and BP should be kept below 130/90 mmHg. In most patients with diabetes it is found that two or more antihypertensive agents are required to achieve the target BP control.

Uncontrolled BP affects adversely

A person with high BP must get it treated and controlled as this disease could put the person into a great health risk. The health problems that may surface are:

- cardiovascular diseases-as angina, stroke, heart attack
- kidney damage
- damaged sight

The high blood pressure could damage the blood vessels in the kidney, which could mean that wastes and excess fluid does not get removed. The excess fluid will increase the blood pressure and over time if a person does little to lower the blood pressure through diet and medication, it may lead to kidney failure.

This causes a condition called *nephrosclerosis.*

OTHER CAUSES

Kidney failure, kidney's problem

Primary reasons are inherent problems with the kidney and could at times be genetic. It may be noted that an individual has no control over the disease and its progress. Hence it is a natural consequence of the state of the organ. Some of these include:

- Glomerular nephritis
- IgA Nephropathy
- Polycystic kidney disease
- Alport syndrome
- Reflux nephrology
- Kidney stones and infection
- Chronic interstitial nephritis
- Renal vascular CKF
- Vasculitis

- Kidney Cancer
- Lupus

  There are many other very rare diseases like Atypical hemolytic uremic syndrome (aHUS), Neurogenic bladder, Spina Bfida, Primary hyperoxaliuria, Hypophosphatemic rickets and new conditions are emerging each day.

Glomerular nephritis

This is one of the most common causes. Diseases may affect kidney function when they attack the glomeruli *[tiny units in the kidney that clean blood]*. Glomerular diseases could be due to genetic or environmental causes, but they largely belong to two categories:

- Glomerulonephritis is an inflammation of the membrane tissue *[which acts as a filter, separates the waste and extra fluid from the blood]*
- Glomerulosclerosis is when tiny blood vessels in the kidney gets scarred or hardened

Both these conditions lead to kidney failure. Majority of cases are due to formation of antibodies to glomeruli or filtering of antigen-antibody complexes by glomeruli.

The diseases damage the *glomeruli* and in the process some protein and red blood cells leak into the urine. The kidneys normally clear the waste products. Sometimes this filtration may be affected so that waste gets left in the blood. The loss of blood protein like albumin means a fall in the level of albumin in the blood. Albumin plays a vital role in absorbing extra fluid from the body into the bloodstream, till the kidney finally removes extra fluid. Due to the lower level of albumin, the capacity to absorb the excess fluid is reduced. Excess fluid gets retained which could lead to swelling in the face, hands, feet, or ankles.

Common signs of glomerular disease

Before being checked up by a doctor, *glomerular* disease can be detected if:

- The urine is frothy, indicating high levels of protein in the urine
- The urine is pinkish in colour, which could be blood in the urine-
- There is swelling in parts of the body - *edema*

The blood tests could reveal-

- Low blood protein, in medical terms-*hypoproteinemia*
- High levels of creatinine, urea and nitrogen in the blood indicate that the kidney's capacity to filter waste is affected, which is known as - *reduced glomerular filtration*

Urine analysis could show-

- High levels of protein - *proteinuria*
- Blood in the urine - *hematuria*

If both the blood and urine tests show some signs of the above problems, a *renal imaging* – ultrasound or x-ray may be recommended. Other than this a kidney biopsy may help in confirming the *glomerular* disease and identifying the exact reason for the disease.

Known causes of glomerular disease

There are a number of different diseases that could result in swelling or scarring of the nephron or glomerulus leading to glomerular disease. It could be due to an infection, drug that harms kidneys, a disease like *diabetes* or *lupus* that affects the entire body. Sometimes glomerular disease can occur without reason or associated with any disease.

IgA nephropathy

Many names have been derived from the description of kidney changes observed on kidney biopsy over three decades but IgA nephropathy is the name commonly used. Berger's disease has been often used in the past to describe the currently known IgA nephropathy. Berger's disease was named after a French pathologist Jean Berger who first reported seminal observations in Paris in the late 1960s.

IgAN is the response of the your immune system to viruses. This response affects the kidneys. When the body is attacked it releases *Immunoglobulin A (IgA),* a protein that helps the body fight infections. Sometimes the IgA protein gets stuck in the kidneys resulting in an inflammation. Due to inflammation one observes blood (hematuria) and protein (proteinuria) in the urine. It needs a biopsy to confirm the disease.

IgA is a most often a slowly progressive disease so people can manage the disease for a long time, though in some people it grows aggressively leading to a kidney failure. Some instances have been found where the disease has affected a cluster of families. There could be genetic factors playing a role in spreading the disease.

Polycystic kidney disease

Polycystic kidney disease (PKD) is a genetic disorder. It is caused due to cysts in the kidney which are water filled. PKD cysts enlarge the kidneys, thereby replacing much of the normal structure, resulting in reduced kidney function and leading to kidney failure.

After a few years in cases when PKD results in a kidney failure, the person will require dialysis or kidney transplantation. In people with the most common PKD, about half the people have a kidney failure.

The PKD can cause cysts in the liver and create problems for blood vessels in the brain and heart. To determine if this is a case of

PKD or a simple cyst, information on the number of cysts and the complications they cause is sufficient.

Alport syndrome

Alport syndrome, the second most common inherited cause of kidney failure, usually affects young men. It can affect older people and women, too.

In each kidney there are one million tiny filtering units (glomeruli) and blood is filtered across the glomerular basement membrane (GBM). In Alport syndrome, one of the proteins that make up the GBM is absent or abnormal. The GBM looks normal in childhood, but deteriorates with time because it lacks the special protein. This leads to kidney failure. This basement membrane is also found in the inner ears and in parts of the eyes, which could lead to deafness and eye problems.

Alport syndrome is much more common in boys and men as the gene that usually causes it (called COL4A5) is on the X chromosome. Men have only one X chromosome, while women have two X chromosomes (XX), so women usually have a normal copy as well as an abnormal copy of the gene.

Women who carry the disease may have minor kidney trouble, such as blood or protein in the urine, sometimes with high blood pressure, but occasionally get severe disease and develop kidney failure. The lifetime risk of severe kidney disease for women who carry Alport's may be as high as 1 in 5, but most never get severe trouble, and those who do are usually much older than men who are affected.

Chronic interstitial nephritis

When the spaces between the kidney tubules get swollen or inflamed they could affect the kidney's ability to filter the waste products. This condition is called interstitial nephritis. If this is a short term condition it is acute and it may become worse and develop into a chronic condition.

Some of the causes for interstitial nephritis could be:

- Drug allergies
- Analgesic nephropathy caused by damage to the kidney due to prolonged medication of pain relievers
- Effects of certain antibiotics
- Medications such as nonsteroidal anti-inflammatory drugs (NSAIDs), furosemide, and thiazide diuretics could produce the condition

When it becomes severe it is likely to be chronic and damage the kidney, particularly in elderly patients.

Some symptoms that may be noticed are:

- Blood in the urine
- Change in volume of urine output
- Change in mental condition like feeling drowsy or confused
- Feeling of nausea
- Rashes
- Swelling
- Weight gain due to fluid retention

Renal vascular CRF

The renal vascular CRF occurs due to some large vessels have abnormalities. If a renal artery is narrowed due to stenosis, the large arteries are unable to supply adequate blood to the kidneys for its functioning. This leads to the elevated blood pressure resulting in hypertension. Insufficient blood supply could shrink the kidney and result ultimately in a CRF.

Vasculitis

This is an inflammation of the small blood vessels and covers many uncommon diseases involving the vascular system. In vasculitis the inflammation damages the walls of various blood vessels. A certain pattern is involved in distribution of blood vessel and how they reach particular organs and through tests abnormalities are revealed. The organ that will be affected by the blood vessel is determined by which organ is reached by the blood vessel and in the process the organ will be damaged. As a group, these diseases are referred to as vasculitides.

Kidney Cancer:

Renal cancer (kidney cancer) is caused by kidney's cell becoming cancerous and growing into a tumor. In most people the kidney cancers is seen in the lining of kidney's tiny tubes (tubules). Most of the kidney cancers get detected they metastasize to distant organs. Early detection is always, easier to treat successfully. However, these tumors could grow large before it is discovered.

First reported in 1826, scientists have yet to discover the cause of renal cancer. Kidney cancer occurs most often after the age of 40; however, children as young as six months have also been diagnosed. Kidney cancer affects almost twice as many men as women. It also tends to be somewhat more common in African American men than white men.

Overall, the lifetime risk for developing kidney cancer is about 1 in 63 (1.6%).

Lupus

Lupus as a disorder was noticed in three periods, classical, neoclassical and modern. The disease was recognized in the

Middle Ages, i.e. the classical period as a classic malar rash and was referred to as lupus, a description given by the 12th century physician, Rogerius. The neoclassical period began in 1872 with Móric Kaposi's revealing the systemic manifestations of the disease. Discovery of the LE (lupus erhythematosus) cells in 1948 heralded the modern period. LE cell, however, is also found in other conditions. The disease is now characterized by advances in the knowledge of the pathophysiology, a clinical and laboratory features, and treatment.

The condition

Lupus nephropathy or systemic lupus erythematosus (SLE) is a rheumatic disease that has autoantibodies directed against self-antigens, immune complexes formation, and immune dysregulation. The disease's manifestations are adequately explained by its name. *Systemic* describes the capability of the disease to affect many organs or systems in the body, involving both internal and external parts of the body. The rash that appears with the onset of the disease covers the cheeks and the nose bridge. This coverage reminded the doctors of the wolf's white patch on its face and since in Latin the word for wolf is *lupus*, the disease got its name. Lastly, *erythematosus* means red in Latin, which is colour of the skin rash brought out by lupus.

The illness is recognized as being unpredictable, with patients exhibiting symptoms or being affected by the acute life-threatening disease. Due to its protean manifestations, lupus should be diagnosed by its differing conditions, such as fevers whose origin cannot be established, anemic condition, some type of nephritis, psychosis, arthralgia, and even fatigue. Patients diagnosed early hence receiving treatment for their symptoms, have helped in prognosis of a disease that was earlier considered as fatal.

The disease affects the immune system, which has millions of white blood cells that protect the body from foreign invasions such as bugs or germs thereby guarding against infections. The white blood cells are grouped in accordance with specific tasks assigned in fighting invaders or foreign antigens. A population of cells called monocytes, have capability of recognizing foreign antigens and send alerts to the T cells or T lymphocytes, who help in fighting the antigens. In turn the T cells send message to the B lymphocytes that produce the antibodies that overpower the antigens by attaching to them.

The cells eat up the antigen/antibody complexes thereby cleaning up the mess. When sufficient antibodies are produced to encounter the antigens, further production of antibodies are stopped by a signals sent to Suppressor T cells, that is another group of T cells, finally the communication is received by B cells to stop the production activity. In the healthy immune system, things return to normal until the next time the person gets sick.

The symptoms and the causes

In a condition of the person with lupus, the immune system does not work properly for unidentified reason. The antibodies produced by B cells, attack the antigens, but the antigens in this case are not foreign invaders but parts of the person's body, cell or tissues. So a person diseased by lupus makes auto antibodies that react with self-antigens and these two combine to make immune complexes.

Cells assigned with the cleaning task, cleans up the immune complexes circulated by the blood. But over time cleaning immune complexes becomes a huge challenge and the cells tire with the activity. The immune complexes travel with the blood vessels and on the way it gets deposited at some point in the body. As a result different parts of the body like skin, hair, joints may become sick with lupus or get inflamed.

In lupus, if parts of the body are affected it will become hot, red, swollen and sometimes tender. Painful and swollen joints showing existence of arthritis, red skin indicating a rash, hair loss meaning alopecia, hands changing colors in the cold, which is the Raynaud's phenomenon and mouth sores, are symptoms of the disease. In spite of the discomfort and pain these symptoms cause, they do not bring serious harm to the body's functions and can be treated by medications. In children and adolescents it could involve internal organs making the problem more serious.

If the kidneys get inflamed in children it could develop into nephritis. For those whose brain is affected they may have seizures, serious mood changes or hallucinations. In others it could mean fluid around the heart or lungs. It is clearly important to prevent the internal organ to be affected by lupus and to achieve that, regular visits to the doctor for evaluations such as blood and urine tests is mandatory.

In the early stage when only blood tests show abnormality, treatment for lupus is much easier than later when one or more organs has inflamed, requiring more medications. Most children and adolescents get the warning signs early in the blood tests making early treatment possible.

Clinical Manifestations:

RENAL:

In an unselected group of lupus patients 30-50% may exhibit urine and kidney abnormalities. However, 80% of children and 60% of adults may subsequently develop overt kidney disease. Development of nephritis in patients who developed lupus after the age of fifty years is very uncommon with < 5% being affected.

All lupus patients with kidney disease tend to loose protein in the urine, with significant number of them showing microscopic hematuria, which means blood loss in the urine. These patients also have decreased kidney function and many may be amongst those losing kidney functions rapidly. Hypertension is not seen higher in lupus patients with kidney inflammation but it is more common in those with severe disease. Bladder involvement is also prominent. However, in cases of early recognition and management of SLE, end-stage renal disease develops in < 5% of patients.

Extrarenal:

SLE is a disease known as "the great imitators" because it often mimics or is mistaken for other disorders. The symptoms of SLE vary considerably, appear and disappear, unpredictably. Diagnosis can be confusing and some people suffer unexplained features of this disorder for years without treatment.

Common initials symptoms include fever, malaise, fatigue, muscle pain, and temporary loss of cognitive function. Other features emerge as manifestations of the body organs when involved.

Though 65% may develop skin disease at some point or the other, 30% cases will have skin involvement of which 30% to 50% exhibit typical butterfly rash on the face. Some develop red scaly patches on the skin. Hair loss; mouth, nasal and vaginal ulcers may also be observed in these patients.

The patients commonly seek medical attention for joint pain. All joints may be affected but small joints of hands and wrist are usually affected. It is believed that > 90% of lupus patients develop joint/or muscle pain at some point during the course of this disorder. Lupus arthritis is generally less disabling and does not lead to destructive arthropathy. However, SLE is associated with an increased risk of bone fractures in relatively young women.

Anemia and iron deficiency may develop in greater than 50% of cases. Low platelets and white blood cell counts may result from lupus itself or from the drugs used to treat lupus.

Lupus patients may be accompanied by inflammation of the heart covering, heart muscle and heart valves. Usually mitral valve and tricuspid valves are usually affected and involvement is characteristically noninfective. Atherosclerosis is often present and progresses rapidly compared to general population.

The involvement of the lungs include inflammation of the lung covering (pleura), fluid accumulation in the pleural cavity, lupus pneumonitis, chronic interstitial disease, pulmonary hypertension, pulmonary emboli, pulmonary hemorrhage, and shrinking lung disease.

Lupus can affect both central and peripheral nervous systems. The diagnosis of neuropsychiatric involvement in this disorder present a great challenge in medicine, as it may have so many patterns of symptoms, some of which may mimic an infectious process or stroke. The most common symptom is headache and other manifestations include cognitive dysfunction, seizures, anxiety and mood disorders, cerebrovascular disease, polyneuropathy, and psychosis. The intracranial pressure may increase with attendant complications. Many other neuropsychiatric complications are rarely observed in SLE.

Treatment:

The treatment of SLE involves preventing flares and reducing their severity and duration when present. It includes corticosteroids and antimalarial drugs. Renal involvement requires different cytotoxic depending on the histologic changes, severity of disease, and renal function.

Sunlight is known to exacerbate the disease and should be avoided. Occupational exposure to silica, pesticides and mercury may also make the disease worse.

Transplantation:

There may be conflicting results. Generally, there is no difference in graft survival and patient mortality compared to non-lupus transplant recipients after first cadaveric and living-related kidney transplant. The reported rates of recurrence are also widely variable; however, recurrence with graft failure occurs at a rate comparable to all the allograft transplants and accounts for less than 4%.

Spread of lupus by population

Today, the rate of lupus varies between countries, influenced by ethnicity, and by gender. As far as rise in its incidence, it is unclear if it can be attributed to better diagnosis or to increasing frequency of the disease.

In the US, the prevalence of SLE is estimated at 53 per 100,000, translating to about 159,000 out of >300 million people, while in Northern Europe it has captured lives of almost 40 out of every 100,000 individuals. The rate is much higher in Afro-Caribbean descent and reaches as high as 159 per 100,000.

Comparing the disease's behavior among African Americans and Caucasians, it has been observed that the former have a threefold increased incidence of lupus as they develop the disease at a younger age, with earlier setting-in of nephritis and, with higher mortality rate. There is a tendency of SLE to impact more lives and with far greater severity in people of non-European descent. This is true also for Hispanics and Asians who also face severe nephritis compared to Americans. Recent studies show higher proportion of lupus patients receiving dialytic therapy for chronic kidney disease. Mortality outcome in lupus patients receiving dialysis is not different from the overall dialysis patient population.

Like many autoimmune diseases, it is primarily a disease of young women, with the incidence at its peak between the ages of 15-40 years. However, it can be found among people of all ages, infants to advanced ages. The female: male ratio rises from 2:1 in pre-pubertal children, up to 4.5:1 in adolescents to 8:1 in adult, and decreasing to 2:1 in patients over 60 years of age. While the estrogen hormone in females seems to be a precipitating factor in the emergence of lupus, in males their hormone, androgens plays a protective role so much so lupus does not favor the male gender.

Another interesting aspect about lupus is that it appears to display familial aggregation, with higher prevalence among first-degree relatives. In monozygotic twins SLE occurs concordantly in as high as 25% to 50% while only 5% of dizygotic twins share the condition. In extended families, this disease may be associated with other autoimmune disorders such as hemolytic anemia, thyroiditis, and idiopathic thrombocytopenia purpura. However, most cases of the SLE are sporadic.

Dr Mohammad Akmal

CKD - MANAGEMENT, ISSUES AND TREATMENTS

Hyperparathyroidism: Hyperparathyroidism is a common complication of chronic kidney disease. The increase in parathyroid hormone generally follows the decline in the kidney function. Parathyroid gland regulates calcium levels in the blood and hyperparathyroidism is caused due to improper calcium regulation. Four pairs of parathyroid glands are situated behind the thyroid glands to monitor and controls calcium in the blood and bones by secreting parathyroid hormone (PTH).

Hyperparathyroidism occurs when one or more parathyroid glands enlarge or develop into a tumor. And subsequently, it releases large quantities of parathyroid hormone that enters the blood. Excess hormone goes through the blood into bones and activates cells in the bone that eat away the bone and multiple complications associated with excess parathyroid hormone develop. Dietary phosphorous restriction, vitamin D and vitamin like agents and specific therapy may arrest or reverse this condition. In some cases surgical removal of 2/3 of glands may be needed.

Hyperphosphatemia (high levels of phosphorous) is common particularly in late stages of CKD. As CKD advances, phosphorous regulation and loss of phosphorous via kidney are lost and hyperphosphatemia develops. Observational studies have determined that hyperphosphatemia is an independent cardiovascular risk factor in CKD. Mechanistically, it has been suggested that it has direct stimulus to vascular calcification. Cardiovascular calcification contributes to extreme mortality in CKD. Dietary restriction and phosphate binders are used to control phosphorus levels in the blood.

Problems created by excess phosphorus, calcium and heightened parathyroid: The blood level of parathyroid hormone plays a critical role in controlling calcium and phosphorous levels. This complex complication results from many factors and high phosphorous plays a pivotal role in inducing hyperparathyroidism. The multiple complications may affect organs like-heart, bones, brain, blood cells and skin etc.

In **Lucy's case hyperparathyroidism caused

- Enlarged heart with poor function
- Very high phosphorous and calcium problems meant calcium deposition in tissues and bone abnormalities developed
- In both shoulders she had large ball like abnormalities
- Combination of her conditions made it inevitable for parathyroidectomy to be conducted, by removing 3 ½ of her parathyroid glands.
- Next step was resolving calcium deposition around her shoulders.

Hyperparathyroidism begins to develop when kidney function is about 60% and is almost a universal finding in dialysis patients. It is associated with damage to many tissues and organs in the body in dialysis patients. As the kidney fails significantly there is reduced production active vitamin D by the kidney and development of hyperphosphatemia. To simplify, these factors directly stimulate the production of parathyroid hormone as well as indirectly by causing reduction in blood calcium. Hyperphophatemia in addition to many complications in CKD also contributes cardiovascular disease.

Tuberculosis: TB peritonitis is uncommon but unusual features like night sweats, weight loss, unexplained fevers should be attended particularly in PD patients from countries with TB endemics and patients with poor immune system like AIDS.

Hepatitis C: Overall, the incidence in the world is 3.3 %. Long-term infection with hepatitis C(HCV), known as chronic hepatitis C is usually a silent infection for decades until liver is significantly damaged by the virus resulting in signs and symptoms of liver disease. Chronic hepatitis begins with an acute phase, which usually goes undetected as it rarely leads to symptoms. If symptoms develop, they may include jaundice, nausea, fever, and muscle aches. Acute phase appears one to three months after the exposure to the virus and last two weeks to three months. Acute phase may not become chronic and in about in 14-50 % there is spontaneous viral clearance and it is also responsive to antiviral therapy.

The infection spreads when contaminated blood enters the blood of an infected person. Worldwide, HCV exists in several forms known as genotypes. Type 1 is more common in North America and Europe but presence of type 2 is less common. These two types are found throughout the world. However, other genotypes cause infection in the majority of patients in the Middle East, Asia and Africa. Even though chronic hepatitis C runs a similar course regardless of the genotype but treatment varies depending on genotype.

Risk factors are as follows:

1. A health care worker exposed to infected blood, which could occur if skin is pierced by an infected needle
2. Injected or inhaled illicit drugs
3. Persons with HIV infection
4. Tattoo piercing with an unsterile equipment
5. Blood transfusion and organ transplantation before 1992
6. Transfusion of clotting factor concentrates before 1987
7. Long –term Hemodialytic therapy
8. Infant born to a hepatitis C infected woman
9. History of being ever in prison
10. The highest incidence in people born between 1945-1965.

Complications: After 20-30 years of hepatitis C, liver cirrhosis and advanced liver failure may occur. Liver cancer may develop in small number of cases. It is also associated with many extrahepatic manifestations that include; impaired glucose metabolism, cryoglobulinemic vasculitis, B-cell non-Hodgkin lymphoma and chronic kidney disease. The membranous and membranoproliferative glomerulonephritis and cryoglobulinemia induced vasculitis are other significant associated medical conditions.

Diagnosis and treatment: It is diagnosed with special MRI, special ultrasound and biopsy. Antiviral treatment used at appropriate time is very effective. Transplantation in appropriate cases is also offered.

Hepatitis B: It is highest in Western Pacific Region and Africa with > 6% of the adult population. The prevalence in Eastern Mediterranean Region 3.3 %, South East Asia 2.0 %, European Region 1.6 % and in 0.7 % of Americas is found.

The renal disease most commonly associated with hepatitis B (HBV) infection include; membranous nephropathy, membranoproliferative glomerulonephritis and polyarteritis nodosa. Hepatitis B can also cause cirrhosis of liver, liver failure and cancer.

It spreads when people come in contact with the blood, open sores and body fluid of someone with hepatitis B virus. In most cases disease does not last a long time, as body fights off the infection within a few months and the person becomes immune for the rest of life.

Some people fail to get rid of the infection and if it lasts for more than 6 months, they become carrier, even if they are symptoms free and are able to transmit the disease to others.

Diagnosis is made with blood test for hepatitis virus and liver biopsy if disease becomes chronic.

Treatment: If patient is exposed to the virus within two weeks, consult a doctor who will give a vaccine and hepatitis B immune globulins that will immune system and fight off the infection. Patient will be advised against alcohol consumption and acetaminophen ingestion. Early recognition and appropriate antiviral therapy may reduce liver cirrhosis, liver failure and cancer.

Multiple myeloma: Multiple myeloma was known to the world as early as 1844 when Samuel Solly reported a well-documented case. A few years later, a London trader, Alexander McBean was found to be excreting a large amount of protein. In 1847 Henry Bence Jones, a physician and chemist identified a globulin protein, suggesting it as multiple myeloma. Thereafter this protein was referred to by his name.

Magnesium: Magnesium is as an essential metal needed in many functions of human cells. The kidney plays very important role in magnesium metabolism. Magnesium is the second-most abundant intracellular cation and, overall, the fourth-most abundant cation. It plays a fundamental role in many functions of the cell, including energy transfer, storage; protein, carbohydrate, and fat metabolism; maintenance of normal cell membrane function; and the regulation of parathyroid hormone (PTH) secretion. Systemically, magnesium lowers blood pressure and alters peripheral vascular resistance. It is also a naturally occurring crystal inhibitor and plays a role in preventing kidney stones.

The average body content of magnesium is 25 gram and 60 % is found in bone, 20 % in muscle, and remaining 20 % in soft tissue and the liver. About 99 % of total body magnesium is in the cells and bone dependent and 1 % is outside the cells.

In advanced chronic kidney disease blood levels of magnesium are increased. On the other hand, low levels of magnesium may result insulin resistance, diabetes, hypertension, atherosclerosis and inflammation. These factors play a major role in the progression of chronic kidney disease. Moreover, low level of magnesium has been associated with cardiovascular disease and all-cause mortality in end-stage renal disease (CKD). Low magnesium levels may also lead to decline in kidney function in CKD and poor function and survival of the kidneys in kidney transplant patients. How low magnesium level causes these abnormalities is not known. Further studies are needed in chronic kidney disease and dialysis patients for clarification. However, studies suggest that high magnesium levels and magnesium supplementation may reduce vascular calcification in CKD.

Abnormalities of magnesium levels, such as hypomagnesemia (low blood levels magnesium), can result in disturbances in nearly every organ system and can cause potentially fatal complications (e.g., arrhythmia, coronary artery vasospasm, hypertension, coronary artery disease, nerve and muscle damage, osteoporosis, diabetes and kidney stones. It is also associated with many other miscellaneous conditions (e.g., migraine, asthma, chronic fatigue syndrome, sudden death in athletes, and sudden infant death etc) secondary to poorly understood mechanism

Despite the well-recognized importance of magnesium, low and high levels have been documented in ill patients, as a result of which, magnesium has occasionally been called the "forgotten cation." It is also a naturally occurring crystal inhibitor and plays a role n preventing kidney stones.

The factors that control magnesium metabolism are absorption from the gut and loss in the urine. The average American diet contains about 360 mg of magnesium. Magnesium is abundantly found in green vegetables, cereal, grain, nuts, legumes and chocolate. Vegetables, meats fish and fruits contain intermediate quantities. The magnesium content is severely decreased by cooking and food processing and thus a large segment of population consume less than required normal allowance.

Magnesium is principally absorbed in small intestine. Absorbed. In normal circumstances 30-40 % magnesium is absorbed and under conditions of low magnesium intake higher percentage is absorbed depending on the amount of magnesium ingested.

The risk of hypomagnesemia can be summarized as follows:

- 2% in the general population
- 10-20% in hospitalized patients
- 50-60% in intensive care unit (ICU) patients
- 30-80% in persons with alcoholism
- 25% in outpatients with diabetes

One reason oxalate is not usually readily absorbed from the gut is that it is complexed with calcium, to a large degree. Ordinarily, little fat reaches the colon. However, in fat malabsorptive states, fatty acids reach the colon and bind calcium, thus freeing up oxalate for absorption. Bile acid malabsorption might also contribute by inuring intestinal cells and increasing colonic permeability. Common causes of enteric hyperoxaluria include the now jejunoileal bypass, as well as modern bariatric procedures, patients with inflammatory disease like Crohn's disease and intestinal resection.

Hemodialysis: For millions of the patients with end-stage renal disease worldwide (CKD 5, ESRD), hemodialysis has become a routine therapy. This life saving therapy has only be applied for > than 40 years. The commonest cause of end-stage renal disease is diabetes followed by hypertension.

The highest prevalence rate for ESRD is found in Japan at 2045 per million, followed by United States with a rate of 1509 per million population. 52% of global dialysis population resides in Japan, USA, Germany and Brazil that make11% of world population.

A recurrent controversy involving the question whether peritoneal or HD represents a superior therapy. This is a difficult question to answer with certainty because selection of two treatments is biased and not random. In general, patient selected for PD have less comorbid conditions independent of other factors that may influence modality selection.

Among the accepted criteria for initiating dialysis are creatinine clearance are 15 mL/min for diabetics and 10 L/min for nondiabetics.

The following factors improve the morbidly and mortality; adherence to the prescribed dietary and fluid restriction, BP control, appropriate correction of anemia, control of calcium, phosphorus and hyperparathyroidism, control of hyperlipidemia, cardiovascular monitoring, adequacy of dialysis, control of diabetes in diabetics, prevention of infection and intradialytic hypotension.

Hypotension: It is the most common acute complication of HD occurring in approximately 20-50% of the dialytic treatments. A greater number of episodes are encountered in older patients and women. Drop in BP during dialysis treatment especially when it occurs frequently is associated with an increased morbidity and mortality. Dialysis procedure is considered to be of two separable procedures, convection and diffusion.

Convection refers to the movement of fluid and solute brought by pressure across the dialysis membrane (transmembrane pressure). Higher the transmembrane pressure, greater the movement of fluid and solute across the dialysis membrane.

The process of fluid removal by the hydraulic force is termed ultrafiltration UF0. During an isolated UF, a progressive increase in total systemic vascular resistance maintains BP as fluid is removed. When diffusion is added to UF (usual dialysis treatment, combination of UF and diffusion), thermal energy can be transferred from heated dialysis to the patient resulting in vasodilatation and increased flow to the skin. As a result, vasoconstriction becomes less effective and maintenance of central blood volume may be impaired when fluid is removed. Cardiac output and BP are maintained by heart rate and in some instance by an increase in myocardial contractility. Unfortunately, when intravascular volume is low, aforementioned two factors may fail to maintain a tolerable BP. Further more the significant heart disease in dialysis patients often limits the ability of the heart and the vessels to appropriately respond to the stress of fluid removal. Impaired autonomic function in these patients also limits the reflex vasoconstriction response during hypotensive episodes.

Very large intradialytic weight gain cannot be easily removed during a typical treatment (3.5-4 hours), even in the presence of fluid overload, as refilling of intravascular space is time dependent. Hypotension in these patients is an exponential function of the rate of fluid removal, especially if removed in excess of 1.5 L/hr. Hypotension can occur in dialysis patients who are at or below estimated dry weight when volume shifts no longer are able to compensate for intravascular depletion and maintain BP. Estimated dry weight is defined as that weight below which the patient develops symptomatic hypotension in the absence of edema and excessive weight gain during dialysis.

Other factors that may contribute to hypotension include; antihypertensive medications, low hematocrit, arrhythmias, poor cardiac function, pericardial effusion, sepsis, and inappropriately larger size of dialyzer.

Management: First step is to determine whether it occurs early or late in the treatment. If it occurs late in the treatment in a patient who was previously stable and free from edema and heart failure, the likely cause will be underestimated estimated dry weight. Therefore, reducing the UF during dialysis, and by effective raising dry weight after dialysis will correct the hypotension. In contrast, the patient who gains excessive weights between dialysis may become hypotensive early in treatment before dry weight is achieved because the rate at which fluid can be mobilized to refill the intravascular space is limited. These patients are required to limit excessive weight gains between dialysis, and increase in frequency and duration of treatment. Specific management of aforementioned factors will also be needed.

Hypotension when occurs, is treated by placement of the patient in Trendelenburg position, administration of 100-200 ml normal saline bolus, and reduction of UF, at least temporarily. Other alternative treatments are with mannitol, glucose, hypertonic saline and albumin. In some individuals, supplemental oxygen may be useful to improve hypoxemia and cardiac contractility.

Infection: It is the second leading cause of death in HD patients and responsible for mortality rate of 12-22%. Septicemia accounts for 75% of these infections. Overall, the annual percentage of mortality resulting from sepsis is 100 to 300 fold higher than in general population. Dialysis access is an important risk factor and using a catheter is at much higher sepsis risk compared to the dialysis access.

Fever in dialysis patient should alert the physician to the strong possibility of infection

Muscle Cramps: It second most common reported complication of HD occurring in as many as 20% of dialysis treatments. Pathogenesis remains uncertain but appears to be more high, when UF rates are high during hypotension in dialysis, and when dialysate with low sodium concentration is employed, indicating development of cramps caused by extracellular volume contraction.

Reducing UF rates, IV normal saline (200 ml), (50% dextrose in water), or 5 mL may help. The pain from severe cramps may be alleviated by administration of diazepam but there is risk of hypotension.

Quinine sulphate, is effective in preventing cramps if administered 1-2 hours before dialysis. It increases the refractory period and excitability of skeletal muscles. Monitor for development of thrombocytopenia. Vitamin E and carnitine have also been tried with variable effects.

Peritoneal Dialysis: In Germany, Ganter was first to perform peritoneal dialysis (PD in humans in 1920s. However, Palmer developed a catheter made of silicon rubber and used to treat small number of patients with acute renal failure in 1940s. The experience continued to improve and first began to be utilized in patients with chronic end-stage renal failure. Subsequently, pioneers like Tenchhoff and others developed cuffed catheters and automated cycling equipment. Intermittent PD to treat end-stage renal disease had become relatively more common by mid 1970s. Subsequently, it evolved in to a modality utilized to treat thousands of patients after development of continuous ambulatory peritoneal dialysis (CAPD) by Moncrief and Popovich in 1977. With passage of time Oreopoulos and Nolph with his colleagues made further modifications that has facilitated the widespread use of CAPD. Low cost, relatively simple technique and the ease with which it could be used at home by the patient has made it a popular dialysis modality.

PD has seen enormous success for over 30 years, which has been possible by better understanding of human anatomy and physiology essential for this modality and recognition of complications.

Peritonitis: It is a leading cause of complication resulting in increased morbidity, technique failure, hospitalizations and occasionally mortality. Its frequency has decreased over the years because of more awareness and early recognition, improved technique and better preventive measures. It can be caused by gram positive organisms, gram negative organisms, fungi and antitubercular treatment.

Diagnosis: Three cardinal features of peritonitis are cloudy effluent, abdominal pain and a positive effluent culture. Typically, these three are present. However, two of three features are sufficient to make a convincing diagnosis.

- A patient with PD presenting with cloudy effluent is likely to have peritonitis unless proven otherwise.
- Abdominal pain may precede cloudy effluent and intensity of pain varies with the type of organism causing the infection.
- With pseudomonas and fungal peritonitis, pain is generally more severe.
- The presence of high fever is not typical of PD peritonitis and indicates sepsis.
- Effluent should be sent for total and differential WBC, gram stain and blood culture before antibiotic therapy is initiated.
- Effluent WBC > 100 cells/ul and neutrophils > 50 % are suggestive of peritonitis. With proper culture technique effluent should be positive in 80-90 % of peritonitis.
- A negative culture with effluent leukocytosis and suggestive symptoms of peritonitis may indicate fastidious organisms, pre-existing antibiotic therapy, inadequate collection and sample technique, nonbacterial infection or laboratory problems. Repeat culture may become positive. With wide spread use of antibiotics, infection secondary to resistant organisms has become more important.

Management: The important considerations are the initial choice of empiric antibiotic therapy prior to identification of organisms, subsequent choice and duration of therapy depending culture results. Another important question is when and whether to remove PD catheter in severe infections.

Renal Transplantation

Renal transplantation is the treatment of choice for end stage renal disease (ESRD) but unfortunately for a small number of the patients and most of these patients are never evaluated for transplantation. In USA 5 year dialysis mortality is 70%.

Renal transplantation has shown significant improvement in early graft survival and long-term graft function making it more cost effective alternative to dialysis. The transplantation activity in developing countries is poor, with a rate of less than 10 per million population (pmp)in contrast to the developed countries at 45 to 50 (pmp). With an estimated world incidence of end-stage renal disease of 80-110 pop, developed countries fulfill 30-35% of their needs in contrast to 1-2% of developing countries. It has progresses from first kidney transplantation in identical twins in Boston in 1951 to more than 447000 to date.

Before immunosuppression was available renal transplantation was limited to identical twins and majority of the patients with ESRD could not receive transplantation. Since the introduction of immunosuppressive therapy and with continuing improvement in such therapy and effective newer agents there has been a significant impact on both patients and graft survival. Currently, the 1-year patients graft survival rates exceed 90% in most transplant centers in USA.

Although approximately only 25% of adult patients on dialysis and perhaps 95% of pediatric patients with ESRD are referred for transplantation evaluation, the waiting list for kidney transplantation has grown burgeoning large.

With increasing interest in living donation and possibly by utilization of laparoscopic donor nephrectomy in 1994 has resulted not only in substantial growth in living transplant transplants but also in shorter waiting times and improved outcomes.

Some conditions are known to recur in in the transplanted kidney (e.g., IgA nephropathy, oxalises, certain types of glomerular diseases and diabetes). However, the rate of recurrence is low enough to justify transplantation.

There are number of contraindications for renal transplantation, some are to surgery, others for immunosuppression and still others are derived from various concomitant disorders.

Contraindications for surgery include: metastatic cancer, hepatic insufficiency (may be candidates for liver-kidney transplantation), severe cardiac and peripheral vascular disease, serious conditions that are unlikely to improve after renal transplantation, repeated episodes of medical noncompliance and inability to perform rehabilitation adequately after transplantation.

HIV with positive blood test is not a contraindication for kidney transplantation provided that patient has CD4 count is greater than 200/uL for al least for 6 months, undetectable HIV RNA, without any major infections or neoplastic complications, and patient has been stable on antiretroviral therapy for at least 3 months. Adverse effects of immunosuppressive drugs may exacerbate atherosclerosis, hypertension, diabetes, and lipid disorders and therefore, increase cardiac risk after transplantation. Cardiac disease is the most common cause of death in these patients.

Contraindications for immunosuppression are infection and malignancy. Acute infection should be fully resolved at the time of transplantation. In general, one should wait for about 5 years after successful treatment of breast cancer, colorectal cancer, melanoma, diffuse bladder cancer, and non-in-situ ovarian cancer. The risk of recurrence is about 50% if the transplant is performed within 2 years of such treatment, about 35% if it is performed between 2 and 5 years and about only 10%, if it is done after 5 years.

Some tumors may allow shorter waiting list (e.g., nodules of prostatic cancer and focal bladder carcinoma, 1 year (or even less) is reasonable for i-situ uterine carcinoma, some renal renal tumors 9clear cell, Wilms, urothelioma), and basal cell skin carcinoma, no waiting time at all may be reasonable.

The prognosis after kidney transplantation is generally excellent, with 1-year graft survival rates ranging from 90% to 95%. HLA-identical transplants from living related donors have the best graft survival rate, where as transplant from complete mismatch cadaveric donors have the worst.

Post-transplant infections are a major problem in developing countries with 15% developing tuberculosis, 30% cytomegalic problems and nearly 50% bacterial infection.

(Any reference made in the above pages of medicines is only indicative. Please get your medications prescribed through your doctor. Your doctor knows your health better. The above guidance is for your understanding how some issues you could encounter may be handled.)

SAFE PREGNANCY, FOR
PATIENT AND UNBORN

If a patient with chronic kidney disease gets pregnant, it puts both mother and unborn child at high risk. Before conception a patient should discuss the possibility of conception, so physicians could ensure that medications for kidney disease that could have adverse effect on pregnancy and place mother and the fetus in risk is not administered. Appropriate birth control medications for women of childbearing age should be advised.

Patient with chronic kidney disease (Stages 1 and 2), with normal blood pressure and urine with little or no protein in the urine may have normal pregnancy.

Patients with moderate to severe chronic disease (Stages 3-5), the risk of complication is much greater. They need close monitoring during pregnancy.

Pregnancy during dialysis (peritoneal or hemodialysis) is an uncommon event. The risks to mom and fetus are significantly higher. More frequent dialysis, blood pressure and fluid and electrolytes monitoring, and anemia correction are important aspects for a safe delivery. With such measures normal pregnancies have also been reported.

Pregnancy in kidney transplant patients: Pregnancy should be only contemplated in patients who have functioning kidney transplant, stable kidney function and blood pressure, good medical and psychologic condition for more than one year and after detailed discussion with her nephrologist. Certain drugs that will affect kidney function and may have detrimental effects on fetus must be avoided.

Dr Mohammad Akmal

PATIENT CENTRIC ASPECTS: TRAUMA AND NEED FOR SUPPORT

Early challenges:

I recall the first time we left the nephrologist's clinic and were driving home. All of us were quiet. Different people thinking about different aspects! My son was fifteen and ½ years old, he had his own teenage worries. As a mother I was overwhelmed, hence unsure how to tackle such a sensitive subject. It was far easier to remain quiet. But my husband being a practical person with a scientific mind used the ride to seek answers. He made logical assessment of the situation.

Later at home he took the discussions to a different level. It began with making assessment of our son's sad state, emphasizing problems likely to be encountered and all the dangers were laid threadbare enough to let my stomach churn with fear.

All negative aspects of the disease and dangers exposed he talked about alternative way of approaching the subject. How to turn the negatives into positives! Even as these evaluations were happening like a *'mother hen'* I floated around the house as if I was all pervading. Truth was I worried that the teenager was getting so much information that would terrify him!

But I was wrong.

It worked wonderfully. This was a big lesson I learnt about life. Terror shows reason to fight for life. Some people can pull up their sleeve and get to work, while others may hide under the couch.

In life, we need to make a choice. Get into the battlefield and face the adversary, an eye for eye. What transpired in our household that day and few days thereafter gave us the courage to go into the battlefield!

The value of logical thinking will be evident in a short while.

Role of a social worker/ Counselor

Any patient leaving a kidney specialist's room comes out in a state of shock.

If a few others accompany the person, their reactions are similar. From that moment subconsciously a certain clock is ticking inside them spelling death. Irrespective of the person's age and vocation the patient makes the easy choice.

To drown in self pity and stop all activity.

To believe their existence is under threat. (Of course, it is, but it needs to be underplayed!)

To wonder about the value of education or staying employed!

And---To focus only on healthcare!

During the early days they have no capacity to plan and determine their future quality of life. For a mind, lost in the woods... it has lost it's capacity to notice the brightness and warmth of the sun, wonder about the clear blue sky, hear the chirping of the birds, or see the brilliance of the silver stars in the dark of the night... these are nature's elements that could guide them to safety.

They needed *someone* at that early stage to show compassion with an understanding nod, a gentle touch, generate a feeling of dependability! Over time a conversation could build a rapport and draw them into a right approach. Someone who could show them that contemplating any drastic action should actually be placed right at the bottom of their checklist!

Bringing upfront as *"priority"* should be:

- Firstly securing their fort from all dangers, including being driven by their own erratic mind.
- Make a plan for survival.

Ours was something like this.

1. Spent a few hours to understand what had happened! What did we do wrong that landed us in this situation!
2. Find out as much about the disease as possible.
3. Understanding the current stage of the disease and assessing how much time can be 'locked up period' for reaching next stage? Or if we had such power to assess if there is at all any safe period?
4. What is dialysis? What are the types available? How many people survived? This topic is painful as death stares you straight in the eye.
5. How can we get a transplant? What is the success rate? Who can be medically eligible? What are the transplant laws?
6. And, yes importantly the diet!
7. Finance: Where will funds come for this treatment?

All the skeletons were now out of the cupboard. On turning it closely to understand all aspects completely, we were drowned in worry as each one looked scarier, than the earlier one!

Though no 7 is Finance, placed in the last slot as if to say *'money cannot buy everything,'* in the case of chronic kidney disease it ranks *first*. Every kidney patient who doesn't have this commodity feels stranded in middle of a huge deluge. Every rich patient believes he/she can fight CKD with this powerful weapon only to realize that indeed, *"money cannot buy everything!"* Money, money and more money is needed for getting treated and continue living.

Logical thinking can help you confront your fears and control it. Logic is that guide that leads you to enter a clear thinking zone. Death is on the cards for everyone, life is there for people who want and stir in them the *"will"* to survive. The will to survive is very dim but it gathers momentum as you reach another roadblock! One has to tell oneself that it is a delusion and one can be surmounted. One needs to plan how to leap forward.

Back to our way of handling it!

Over the next few weeks, we collected information. My husband made it like a classroom where both my sons were actively participating. I was in hiding. (As a mother my sense of guilt was at its height.) Emotional outbursts were intermittent and my son, who was an exuberant and promising young lad was now spending more time by himself. At odd times he was found surfing the Internet for latest information.

But we made a plan that we followed though with many modifications. On top of the chart, was the unspoken and spoken agenda! To complete schooling, graduate and be on a career path so the future has a smoother road moving in some direction.

Research tells us that a person who continues to be employed is happier.

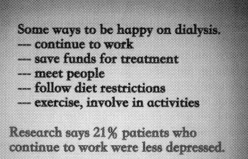

Some ways to be happy on dialysis.
— continue to work
— save funds for treatment
— meet people
— follow diet restrictions
— exercise, involve in activities

Research says 21% patients who
continue to work were less depressed.

You can make a choice.

Vasundhara Raghavan

This above is a sample plan. Make your own survival plan. It can be as exotic as it will be but follow your heart and map your journey to live and with all mental capacities intact.

Airtight plans fail, as we are never sure of the obstacles ahead. But it is also important to break all the walls and try to penetrate. Also, never let our fear build it's own hillock!

But every person has individual mental process for handling a serious disease. So it is important to make your own plan.

Find an outlet for your emotions

Emotional outbursts are a statement of the person's mental state. Let me say it, here now.

It is very much allowed! Go do it.

It is totally permitted to feel the earth slip from under the feet. To feel ruined and that life is at its' natural end. There's no need to say I love life and live under a misguided confidence. That could shatter at the first resistance it faces.

It's almost as if you were in a tunnel and this huge rock blocked the end so no light could penetrate. You have a choice to sit and quietly work on the rock. Your own patience and persistence will never go unnoticed. Slowly chips of the rock will fall at your feet when you hit it, apply pressure. When you're frustrated. Rest. Give vent to your feelings. But go back to doing the only thing possible. Break the barrier.

World respects a person who tried hard! People are amazing when it comes to putting you on a pedestal to worship for your perseverance. Work gets recognized. Courage gets rewarded.

Imagine the total helplessness of a beggar who has only a worn out shirt, with his pocket empty and with hunger gnawing him. He can't see any reason to live. It's like he can see no future at all.

That empty feeling is just what chronic kidney disease awakens in you. One feels cheated as if robbed of something precious. So please feel free to express and yell at the world around you. But after that, calm your nerves. Work on making a resolve to survive.

On the Facebook, a social-media friend Mark Rosen has a special group.

We did a little interaction to understand each person's first reaction to chronic kidney disease. Such a great revelation! So many stood tall in the sands of time, weathering bruises of ego, of body and yet made it to stand testimony of this hour.

Some heart wrenching observations made are:

Joan Gregory said,

> *Shock, some hopelessness and some dread. That was 10 years*

ago. I've stayed around the same numbers since then (Stage 3b). Still it's worrisome!

Virginia Halsey remarked:

> *Charles and I were both scared to death of what would come next!*

Gail Rae-Garwood made a big statement:

> *Terror, abject terror! I thought I was being given a death sentence. Boy, was I ever wrong!*

Dee Moore's speculation tells us how many people could save their kidney!

> *I didn't really think much about it. It happened some 20 years ago. I didn't feel bad, there was no symptom but there was protein in the urine. I knew nothing about creatinine at that time. But today I'm on dialysis, I wonder if I had thought a little bit more about it, met a doctor, would it have been a different situation?*

Patty Powell Oxley's fear was very real...

> *As a newly retired acute care RN, I was scared and felt hopeless. I knew about kidney disease!*

Magda Bonacina's confession speaks a lot:

> *For me: fear... also because nephrologists didn't explain much!*

Mare Daly talks of her husband:

> *Worried and immediately researched to find the best nephrologist in NJ and made an appointment for my*

husband. He's doing great now; battled CKD 18 years, did PD for 2 years and is now 6 months post transplant from our son. Life is wonderful again... Positiveness and not letting this disease define you is key! 🖤 ❤

Mark Rosen, formidable as he is says simply:

FEAR

Jim Bishop tells us a lot:

The kidney disease was diagnosed during a string of heart attacks that led to open heart surgery. I believe the initial reaction was one of being irritated by one more complication.

Lyn Adams Hanlon says,

I was pissed off with my primary doctor. He knew my numbers and said nothing so that I don't worry till I was well into 3rd stage already. Why do they not tell me? It could have been addressed then before it got so far into 4th stage with a GFR of 28.

Sherry Simons tells us about dreams...

For me it was fear. I thought, "I have so much that I still want to do!" But I've realized life is a blessing. I will not give in to my deep fears, yes, it's hard but live each day thankful!

From all this clearly we have something to work on.

1. Talk to your doctor. Get your doubts cleared. Your health is your concern. Doctors have so many patients so busy with other serious cases. You have only your case to deal with. Maintain a good rapport with your doctor. While discussing be a good listener. You will learn many useful things.

2. Talk to your family and friends about your illness. Your sharing how you brushed with kidney disease will guide people with hypertension, diabetes, urinary infection or hematuria and proteinuria. Possible you will save them from reaching ESRD.
3. They may ignore you and call you names. You may be scoffed at, but later if your warning was unheeded and they faced a similar situation they will have only their egos to blame.
4. Be your own master in health matters. Search, find information, and talk to people at the clinic or dialysis center. You will learn to accept your situation; maybe yours will be better compared to theirs.

Need for support:

A person who is already facing a health challenge can show some better sense to catch himself/herself before getting into depression. Once this low mental state sets in, help through counselors must be considered seriously to decrease impact of two major conditions-chronic kidney disease and depression, that could lead to very grave situation.

Counseling is a help given by qualified people who know how to help people retrace steps and find road to survival. However qualified or experienced you may like to choose someone who can understand you better.

Please do your study before you sign up for counseling. Your friends or physician could guide you on this issue.

Being physically and mentally fit to receive for your treatment is important.

Remember this always so you don't miss your opportunity.

> *All of us are important to our families.*
> *We have to keep our intrinsic values one notch higher –*

Keep learning skills, try to work and earn and
Smile through life.
No one cares for a loser.
Winner is not one great successful person.
It is one, who will stand, head held high,
Not in pride but in humility,
CKD is a great teacher of humility,
Humility brings you honor and with it bountiful joy!
See that you keep the fire of love around,
Being your kind self.

Diet for kidney and life:

Be watchful on what you eat based on what you must eat. That's the only way to live. There's no other way. Talk to your doctor and dietician. Their guidance will be of great help. Make your small sacrifices. Leave or limit what is not to be eaten. Better to measure life that is yours and live within the confines. Learn to break those on a rare day – but go back to doing what gave you good health and comfort. CKD is no joke.

Learn to live with knowledge of all essentials.

Exercise:

Like diet exercise is critical for managing all stages of kidney disease. You may discuss with your doctor what is best suited for your condition. Make a regular schedule for exercise. Thereafter try to keep to the schedule.

Vasundhara Raghavan

THE RIDE BEYOND REJECTION!

The rhythm of life is determined by so many celestial controls even as our universe makes its own moves or the waves of the sea change their motion.

Whose kidney goes and whose stays results from the throw of a dice.

Many, people live with their valuable kidney for 20, 30, 40 or even 50years. The dice simply did not select their kidney. Try to tell the aggrieved about this illusive game of dice, it will make sense even if some are more stubborn about their rights. In time understanding will surface that not everyone was meant to be a star.

That said. It's very, very difficult to understand 'the why?' and accept it gracefully. To attain a mastery of that philosophy one has some swallowing to do - of pride, of overwhelming emotion while letting tears flow freely without any inhibition. The anger, the desperateness is an integral part of the game. So there's time needed for the mind to leave the throne and let the heart lead so kneeling meekly in submission of the superior power is possible.

Life can then be picked up piece by piece. Surely no one wants to let anyone tread on scattered pieces of one's self-esteem.

Vasundhara Raghavan

FACING A KIDNEY FAILIRE

By Vasundhara Raghavan

Kidney transplants definitely rank higher than dialysis as a treatment, but in spite of much medical advancement there's a chance of a graft failure.

Research has shown live donor transplants have better survival rates.

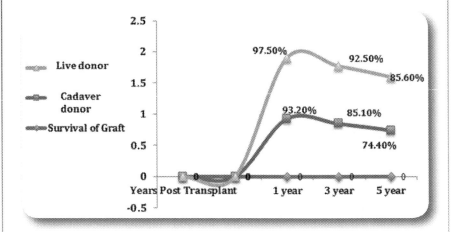

Data used from: Kidney Kaplan-Meier Survival Rates for transplants performed 2008-15. Based on OPTN data as of October 20, 2017. Organ Procurement and Transplantation Network, USA. Chart made by Vasundhara Raghavan.

Live or cadaver transplants, many transplants do fail for several reasons.

- Blood clot: If the blood vessels going to the transplanted kidney has clots formed during the surgery, there is every likelihood the kidney doesn't receive enough blood supply.
- Infections in the kidney can cause serious complications unless identified and treated early.

- In some cases though doctors have recommended the organ for transplant, there could be inherent deep-rooted problems in the kidney that could surface after the transplant. Some of them are treatable while some could create a problem.
- Early rejections must be promptly attended. At some point patient's proactive attention to health care can play a huge role in managing the kidney.

  o Alert to catch signs of infections – cold, cough, fever and taking steps to communicate and meet the doctor
  o Compliance on medications and water in-take. Understanding the concept of a kidney transplant and the role of the immunosuppressant is extremely important. The medications suppress the immune system so the body does not attack the kidney. These are medications are scheduled. So one must be conscious of the timings and take them every day to stay ahead in the *"graft survival game"*.
  o Take simple precautions against infections

- Acute Rejections can be managed with treatments. Though more common in the first few months, it could happen at any time.
- Chronic Rejections means that the kidney is beyond recovery. The kidney is not accepted by the body and is a long-term problem. The kidney will give up in time.
- Some medicines have a tendency of creating a problem to the kidney. These could lead to kidney damage.
- In some instances fluid gets collected around the kidney. If this is not treated in time it damage the kidney.
- Recurrence of the earlier disease. Some diseases that caused the kidney failure could reoccur.

Most often the transplant failure is not due to negligence of the kidney recipient. However, considering how difficult it is to get a transplant, the person must make it a point to:

- Communicate with the nephrologist on small or big issues experienced
- Side effects of medicines could be overcome by some change in medicines
- Be always in control of one's health

Rejection makes another life change

A person who receives a notice, "Your graft has failed!" has to reckon with many aspects of life. However gently this news is delivered, the person's situation cannot be changed. While choosing a transplant the person has been briefed of survival rates of grafts while subtly conveying the 'cons' of a transplant. But reality is what determines the future.

Aftermath of a rejection awakens new perceptions of the future. There is

- Shock – how can this happen?
- Hurt and disappointment surfaces. Some disappointment that the kidney left them early. No matter that it lasted for 5, 10, 20 years but their position has now changed.
- Fear comes back. Fact that life is on a reverse gear means the person goes back to dialysis. A great feeling of insecurity.
- Acceptance that they need to start dialysis. Though most people had a transplant after some dialysis treatments, once they experienced a transplant they need lots of encouragement to get back on dialysis.
- Sadness and frustration to again start registration for a transplant, if it is possible for them.
- Abandoned-During the period that the kidney lasted, people who were strong supporters had moved on in life. There's a new loneliness that envelops them. They need

love, assurance and understanding to be showered. Their file with the Transplant Team is inactive and they need to find new health support. If the rejection has happened with 90 days of transplant, the Transplant Team may request for the person's wait time back.

- Relief... this is experienced by people whose transplant was a very traumatic experience. They may have faced many serious complications, handling many treatments, effects of side effects and multiple hospitalisations. In such a situation it may seem better to stay on dialysis.

Apart from the emotional outbursts, in the first few months there is need to relearn many aspects of the disease that they learnt when first detected is a great challenge.

- Making dietary modifications for hemodialysis
- Getting a fistula in place
- Adapt to rules of the *"Water Game"*

  o Dialysis needed water restriction: of 2 liters of fluid split into 2 days
  o Post Transplant: Consuming 3-5 liters of water each day post transplant (as advised by your transplant physician/nephrologist)
  o Going back on dialysis: 2 liters of fluid over 2 days

Though dietary changes is also a big issue to contend with, this swing in water consumption is most dramatic. In hot climates particularly, water restriction is very difficult. Lots of adjustments are needed to be healthy on dialysis, both emotionally and physically.

Good family, friend, community support will steer the person to rise above the constraints and get registered for a transplant or look for another live donor. It is tough, but not impossible.

It is important for the person whose graft has stopped working to realize how important it is to be alive. Shifting focus on other aspects of health care, looking for alternate dialysis treatments may help in surviving with great positivity.

Glossary of Technical Terms

Access: Access is created for entering the bloodstream so that dialysis can be done. In the case of haemodialysis, a fistula acts as the access.

Acute coronary syndrome: It involves chest pain and other symptoms, when the heart does not get enough blood.

Acute Kidney Injury (AKI): Acute Kidney Failure, AKI is a sudden decline in kidney function. This happens most often due to toxicity of medicines (pain killers and antibiotics), drop in flow of blood caused by severe infections such as sepsis, dehydration and blockage of urine. It will lead to build-up of waste products and create imbalance in electrolytes and body fluids. AKI requires treatment through acute dialysis and is recognized to be associated with greater risk of short-term and long-term death and adverse kidney outcomes.

Albumin is a protein made by the liver. Albumin is found in blood plasma, serum, muscle, the whites of eggs, milk, and other animal substances. A test of blood and urine is done for measuring protein in the blood and urine.

Albuminuria/ Proteinuria: Presence of high albumin or protein in the urine is a sign of some damage to the kidneys. Proteinuria could be result of long-term hyperglycemia (high blood sugar levels) of hypertension (high blood pressure).

Anaemia: If a person feels weak, breathless and less energetic, it may be indicative of being anaemic. When blood has a shortage of red cells, anaemia occurs. For improvement, iron and erythropoietin will be needed.

Angiotensin - converting enzyme inhibitors: This is also known as ACE inhibitors. They are medications for heart that help widen or dilate your blood vessels to improve the amount of blood your heart pumps and lower blood pressure. By increasing blood flow, ACE inhibitors help to decrease the amount of work your heart has to do. Well-controlled blood pressure by some ACE inhibitors has enabled slow progression in kidney damage in many people with type 2 diabetes.

Artery: Artery is the blood vessel that carries blood from the heart to the rest of the body.

Bladder: From the kidney the urine goes into the organ known as the bladder before being released from the body.

Blood cells: The blood is made up of microscopic cells that are known as blood cells. Blood cells consist of red and white cells and platelets.

Blood group: Our blood can be classified into four main groups: A, B, AB, and O. The classification system is based on hereditary conditions dictating the availability of certain antigens in the cells. Generally blood and organ donations are based on the match of blood group between the donor and recipient.

Blood pressure: When the blood passes through the arteries, it exerts a certain level of pressure against their walls. This pressure is measured as blood pressure. Blood pressure is an important determinant for many surgeries and indicates the health condition of a person.

- Normal blood pressure: is 120/80 millimeters of mercury (mm Hg) or less
- Prehypertension: between 120/80mm Hg and 139/89 mm Hg

- High: more than 140/90 mm Hg
- If your age is over sixty-five, blood pressure up to 150/90 mm Hg can be considered normal

Body Mass Index (BMI): An individual's weight in kilograms divided by his or her height in meters squared. It is a measurement of body fat.

Bone marrow: In some bones, such as hip and thigh bones there is a soft tissue in the hollow, interior portion, which is known as bone marrow. New blood cells get created here.

Cadaveric transplant: This is a transplant surgery done with a kidney or other organ removed from a person who is brain dead or has died in an accident.

Calcium: This is a mineral salt that strengthens the bones.

Catheter: A catheter is a flexible plastic tube that is inserted when access to the body's interior is needed.

Cardiovascular: This relates to the heart and the blood vessels involved in blood circulation.

Cholesterol: This is a measure of the level of fat in the bloodstream. There is a risk of having heart diseases or strokes if the blood shows a high cholesterol value. Though high cholesterol is dangerous, the levels can be reduced with diet and drugs.

Creatinine: When muscles are used, a waste substance known as creatinine is produced. A blood test is used to measure creatinine, and it indicates whether or not the kidney is functioning normally.

The normal values for creatinine are: 0.6–1.2 milligrams per deciliter (mg/dL).

Cross match: The cross match is different from tissue type or blood group match. Cross match is a blood test to check for the existence of any antibodies. Antibodies normally help the body fight infection and would react with the donor kidney. High levels of antibodies may lead to rejection, even if it is a good tissue type match.

Cross match is done by mixing a sample of the recipient's blood with cells from the donor. If the recipient's blood starts attacking the donor cells, there is the likelihood that the kidney will be rejected.

Dehydration: The body is dehydrated when there is insufficient water in the body for its proper functioning.

Diabetes: When high levels of glucose are found in the blood and urine, a condition popularly known as diabetes is said to be the problem. This happens because of poor functioning of the pancreas. The world over, people with diabetes are at high risk for kidney failure.

Diabetic nephropathy: Kidney disease that results from diabetes. Diabetic nephropathy is the number one cause of kidney failure. Almost one third of people with diabetes develop diabetic nephropathy at some point unless there is strict control of diabetes through medictions.

Dialyser: A dialysis machine has a filtering unit known as a dialyser, which removes waste products and excess water from the blood.

Dialysis: The process of removing the waste products and excess water from the blood when the kidneys cease to perform this function properly is known as dialysis.

Dietary acid load (DAL): The body's metabolism produces acids and bases of varying levels based on food consumed. The difference between the acids and bases is called the dietary acid load (DAL) or formally, net endogenous acid production (NEAP). These must be buffered or excreted by the body through respiration or urination in order to maintain an acid-base balance.

End-stage renal disease (ESRD): The final stage of kidney failure (as that resulting from diabetes, chronic hypertension, or glomerulonephritis) that is marked by the complete or nearly complete irreversible loss of renal function.[2]

Diuretic drugs: Medicines administered to increase urine outputs are called diuretics.

Donor: A person who donates an organ, blood, or tissue to another person is known as a donor.

Dry weight: The body weight after dialysis is called a dry weight. The weight is without excess fluid in the lungs or in the tissues.

- Dyslipidemia: This condition is marked by abnormal concentrations of lipids or lipoproteins such as cholesterol in the blood.
- Dysrhythmia: This is an abnormal rhythm, especially a disordered rhythm exhibited in a record of electrical activity of the brain or heart.
- Erythropoietin (EPO): When the kidney functions properly, this is a hormone that it produces, along with several others. This hormone stimulates the bone marrow to produce red blood cells. But when the kidney fails, the person may become anaemic if lower levels of red blood cells get produced. In such a situation, EPO injections may be given to perform the hormone's function.

End-stage renal disease (ESRD): When the kidney loses all its functions and reaches the final stage of irreversible loss it has reached ESRD. Such result may be expected from diabetes, chronic hypertension, or glomerulonephritis.

Epidemiology: The study of the distribution and determinants of health-related states or events in specified populations, and the application of this study to control of health problems.

Expanded criteria donor (ECD): Apart from ideal candidates for organ donation now people not considered to be ideal or standard are being evaluated as a possible donor. In this criteria donors that may included are people of advanced ages, with previous infection with hepatitis B or hepatitis C, hypertension or diabetes mellitus, abnormal donor organ function, and non-heart-beating status of a deceased donor.

Fistula: In order to provide access to the bloodstream for haemodialysis, a vein may be enlarged surgically. This access is called a fistula.

Fluid overload: This is excess water in the body caused by excess consumption of water or not being able to pass enough urine.

Glomerular filtration rate (GFR): Glomerular filtration is the process by which the kidneys filter the blood, removing excess wastes and fluids. To determine level of the kidney's functioning a GFR is calculated that shows how well the blood is filtered by the kidneys. That is one way to measure remaining kidney function. GFR is usually a estimation so it is eGFR arrived at by using a mathematical formula that is based on a person's size, age, sex, and race to compare serum creatinine levels.

GFR: how to interpret it

Stage	What that means?	(GFR level)
At increased risk	Kidneys are at risk due to: diabetes, high blood pressure, family history, old age, ethnic group	More than 90
1	Some damage with normal kidney function	90 or above
2	Damage with mild loss of kidney function	89 to 60
3a	Mild to moderate loss of kidney function	59 to 44

3b	Moderate to severe loss of kidney function	44 to 30
4	Very severe loss of kidney function	29 to 15
5	Kidney failure	Less than 15

GFR number tells you at what level the kidney function remains. Your doctor will tell you the stage of kidney disease. GFR goes down with progression of kidney disease.

Information sourced: National Kidney Foundation

Glucose: A sugar found in the blood that is used by cells to produce energy.

Glycemia: The presence of glucose in the blood.

Glycemic control: For people with diabetes, it is important to have a glycemic control which means to have blood sugar at acceptable levels over a prolonged period, usually measured by hemoglobin A1c or fasting blood glucose.

Haemodialysis (HD): A more popular form of dialysis for blood purification. The blood is cleaned outside the body by a dialysis machine, which takes between three and four hours to finish the process.

Haemoglobin: The red blood cells have haemoglobin, which carries oxygen to all parts of the body.

Hemoglobin A1c (HbA1c) test: This test, also called HbA1c, glycated hemoglobin test, or glycohemoglobin, will determine how well diabetes is being controlled. HbA1c gives an average of blood glucose control over a 6 to 12 week period, which along with periodic home blood glucose monitoring is able to appropriately treat diabetes.

Ideal body weight: An ideal body weight is determined based on the age, sex and height of the person. This is the expected range for people falling within that group.

Immune system: Everybody has an immune system that protects the body from infections and foreign bodies. In the case of a person who has had a transplant, the system is suppressed by medication so that it does not reject the foreign organ. The immune system therefore works less effectively.

Immunosuppressant drugs: These are drugs prescribed to transplant patients to make the immune system less effective so that it does not fight the foreign body, which is the transplanted kidney or other organ. Immunosuppressant drugs are required to protect the kidney from being rejected.

Malnutrition: This condition occurs because of weight loss, due to lower consumption of food providing protein and energy.

Macroalbuminuria: Albuminuria is defined as a relatively high rate of urinary excretion of albumin, which could be greater than 300 milligrams per 24-hour period.

Microalbuminuria: Albuminuria is defined as a relatively high rate of urinary excretion of albumin, which could be between 30 milligrams and 300 milligrams per 24-hour period.

Nasogastric tube: This is normally called the NG tube. It is made of a flexible material of rubber or plastic. The tube, used to put substances, including nutrients, into the stomach, is inserted through the nose and then through the esophagus into the stomach when a patient is unable to eat or drink by mouth.

Sometimes the tube is used to remove contents from the stomach, including air, small solid objects, fluid and other toxic substances that cannot be removed normally through the stool.

Nephritis: This is an inflammation of the kidneys.

Nephron: The kidney is made up of many small units called nephrons, which do the filtering and balance fluid in the body.

Oedema: This is an abnormal accumulation of water in the body. If the water is accumulated in the lungs, it is called pulmonary oedema.

Omentum: The omentum hangs like a curtain from the bottom of the stomach, right in front of the intestines. It is like a sheet of fatty tissue that stores body fat, and it grows as more fat is accumulated. It contains germ-fighting cells that can migrate to the abdomen and helps to seal it off. The omentum therefore protects the abdomen from infections. For the surgeon the omentum acts as a handy tool—something like biological duct tape. Portions of the omentum may be used as a graft in cut areas to heal them. The omentum can be also a source of problems. When its blood supply is interrupted, there are symptoms of severe pain and tenderness that can wrongly be diagnosed as appendicitis. Another aspect is that when it is enlarged due to high fat storage, it results in a protruding belly, and the person does not look very pleasing.

Peritoneal dialysis (PD): This form of dialysis uses the peritoneum as a filter. The blood is cleaned inside the person's body, not externally, as in haemodialysis. PD is a home dialysis programme.

Peritoneum: This is a natural membrane lining the walls of the abdomen.

Peritoneal Cavity: This is the area in the abdomen where the stomach, liver, and bowels are found.

Phosphate: An important substance involved with calcium that accumulates when the kidneys fail.

Phosphate binders: In order to avoid the build-up of phosphate in the blood, phosphate binders are prescribed. They absorb excess phosphorus from the blood.

Platelets: These are a type of blood cell that helps in clotting blood.

Polycystic kidney disease: This kidney disease is hereditary and results because of a problem in kidney development. The kidneys get enlarged and are full of sacs filled with fluid, which are known as cysts. This disease sometimes leads to kidney failure.

Potassium: This mineral is normally present in the blood but has to be maintained at a particular level. Higher or lower levels may cause heart problems.

Protein: This is essential for muscle formation, and the breakdown products are filtered by the kidney. Meat, fish, dairy products and nuts are rich in protein.

Proteinuria: The presence of excess protein in the urine.

Pulmonary oedema: When the lungs get filled with fluid, the resulting condition is known as pulmonary oedema. It results in breathlessness, especially when lying down flat and exercising.

Pyelonephritis: This is a painless inflammation caused by repeated infections, drugs, or other factors. It occurs in the part of the kidneys that is in between filtering units.

Recipient: A person who receives an organ for transplant from a donor.

Rejection: The immune system fights infection and foreign bodies. In the case of a transplant, the organ transplanted is in fact a foreign body. The immune system may attack the organ, leading to rejection.

Renal: It is the term used for kidneys. A renal failure means a failure of the kidneys.

Restless Legs Syndrome (RLS): This neurological disorder causes an individual to experience an uncomfortable sensation in his/her legs leading to an urge to move them. Symptoms occur most often at night, as lying down tends to activate the symptoms. The disorder affects both males and females, with a twice a high an incidence in females. With age this syndrome gets worse.

Satellite haemodialysis unit: A unit that is located away from the main hospital renal unit and provides haemodialysis is known as a satellite unit.

Semi permeable: A membrane that allows some substances to pass through it is called semi permeable.

Serum: The fluid portion of the blood obtained after removal of the fibrin clot and blood cells, distinguished from the plasma in circulating blood.

Serum Creatinine: A product of creatinine phosphate that is filtered from blood by the kidneys. Serum creatinine levels rise with decreased renal function

Tenckhoff catheter: In a PD, the catheter that allows access for the dialysis fluid to flow in and out from the peritoneal cavity but is capped off when not in use is known as a Tenckhoff.

Tissue type: A blood test called a tissue type test is conducted to measure the antigens on the surface of the body and its cells.

Transplant: This surgery is done to plant a new organ, which is donated by someone, into a patient who needs it for survival.

Ultra filtration: This process removes excess water from the blood.

Under dialysis: This happens when dialysis treatment is not sufficient to remove all the water and waste products that are in excess.

Urea: This is one of the main waste products that build up in the blood. In addition to creatinine levels, the levels of urea in the blood are indicative of how the kidneys are functioning.

Ureters: Urine is carried from the kidneys to the bladder through tubes called ureters.

Urethra: The tube that carries urine from the bladder outside the body is called the urethra.

Urine: This is the fluid produced by the kidneys. It is composed of excess water and the toxic waste products that come from food and are not required by the body.

Urine protein to creatinine ratio (UPCR): Ratio of urinary protein to creatinine used to quantify the amount of protein being excreted through urine and used to calculate proteinuria

Veins: Blood vessels that carry dark-red–coloured blood are veins. They bring impure blood from different parts of the body to the heart for purification. They have less oxygen and are thinner than arteries.

Bibliography

Listed below are some materials I referenced during the process of writing this book. They helped in my understanding and in providing readers information in simple layman's language. I have attempted to write the book with honesty and as simply as possible.

American Heart Association - www.heart.org/HEARTORG
American Kidney Fund - www.kidneyfund.org
American Urology Association - www.auanet.org
Astellas Transplant - www.transplantexperience.com
Cedar-Sinai Medical Center - www.csmc.edu
Davita - www.davita.com
eMedicineHealth - www.emedicinehealth.com
Healthcommunities.com - www.healthcommunities.com
Kidney School - www.kidneyschool.org
Mayo Clinic - www.mayoclinic.com
MedlinePlus Medical Encyclopedia - www.nlm.nih.gov/medlineplus/encyclopedia.html
MedicineNet.com - www.medicinenet.com
Merriam-Webster Online Dictionary: www.merriam-webster.com
National Kidney Foundation, India - www.nkfi.in
National Kidney Foundation, United States - www.kidney.org
National Kidney Foundation, Southern California - www.kidney.org
National Kidney and Urological Diseases Information Clearinghouse - kidney.niddk.nih.gov/kudiseases
Nephrology Channel - www.nephrologychannel.com
Texas Pediatric Surgical Associates - www.pedisurg.com

The Kidney Foundation of Canada - www.kidney.ca
University of Iowa Hospitals and Clinics - www.uihealthcare.com
University of Pennsylvania Health System - www.pennmedicine.org
WebMD https://www.webmd.com/

Acharya, V. N., "Status of Renal Transplant in India," *Journal of Postgraduate Medicine* (http://www.jpgmonline.com) 40, no.1 (1994): 158-61.

Stein, Andy, and Wild, Janet, *Kidney Dialysis and Transplants*. London: Class Publishing, 2002.

Garovoy, Marvin R., Guttmann, Ronald D, *Renal Transplantation*. New York: Churchill Livingstone Inc., 1986.

Faris, Michie Hall, *When Your Kidneys Fail*. Southern California: National Kidney Foundation, 1994.

Our Gratitude

Through our book, we have connected people with singular goal and purpose. Survive the insurmountable chronic kidney disease. Their experiences were so real and conquest so great that even today they remain in awe that they managed to tame the disease.

Conscious of how inspiration is always needed in huge doses, they agreed to part life experiences so many get encouraged to find their individual treatment goals.

We are forever grateful for this community of people who came together to add value to this book.

Dr Mohammad Akmal
Vasundhara Raghavan

**Kidney disease was never
your choice.**

It just happened.

Love yourself.
Fight to survive.

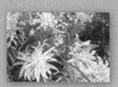

19-02-2017

Printed in the United States
By Bookmasters